This is the best book I've ever read in m
mental health. It advises women how
ing and motherhood, how to weigh al
the most important journey of their life with confidence.

If you are considering breastfeeding your baby, are actually breastfeeding
now, or are providing support for nursing mothers, this book is for you! It
goes beyond the basics to provide the research and tested suggestions needed
to prevent and work with challenges that might occur. Written in a friendly,
positive voice, this is a book which I am excited to highly recommend.

This is the down-to-earth, no-nonsense book we needed about breastfeeding,
and Dr. Kathleen Kendall-Tackett is the researcher, practitioner, and mother
we needed to write it. Equal parts research, science, and practical advice, if
you have questions or concerns about breastfeeding, buy this book!

Kathleen Kendall-Tackett has managed to tackle some of the most common problems facing breastfeeding mothers today and has made them relatable and nonthreatening while providing advice and connecting with the reader not as just an authority but as someone who truly "gets it." It is a book I will be recommending to all new moms so we can once and for all put to bed the idea that breastfeeding has to suck.

—TRACY CASSELS, PHD, DIRECTOR OF *EVOLUTIONARY PARENTING*

An indispensable resource for all new mothers. Kathleen Kendall-Tackett is a trusted expert in the field who uses understandable language to integrate science, her clinical experience, and, crucially, the experiences of mothers. This book cuts through the contradictory messages that new mothers often receive about breastfeeding and provides hope and optimism even in the face of breastfeeding challenges.

—AMY WENZEL, PHD, ABPP, FOUNDER AND DIRECTOR, MAIN LINE CENTER FOR EVIDENCE-BASED PSYCHOTHERAPY, BRYN MAWR, PA

Chapter 2 is pure genius and worth the price of the entire book. In Chapter 2, the "five I's" of new motherhood address contemporary issues that are rarely mentioned in other comparable books: idleness, isolation, incompetence, identity, and intensity. "Mothering is relentless" might be the most insightful phrase in the entire book. The coping strategies in this chapter are brilliantly simple, doable, and practical even if the new mother is alone in her environment.

—LINDA J. SMITH, MPH, IBCLC, BRIGHT FUTURE LACTATION RESOURCE CENTRE LTD.

BREAST FEEDING DOESN'T NEED TO SUCK

BREAST FEEDING DOESN'T NEED TO SUCK

How to Nurture Your Baby and Your Mental Health

KATHLEEN KENDALL-TACKETT, PhD, IBCLC, FAPA

 AMERICAN PSYCHOLOGICAL ASSOCIATION

The opinions and statements published are the responsibility of the author, and such opinions and statements do not necessarily represent the policies of the American Psychological Association.

The author has worked to ensure that all information in this book is accurate at the time of publication and consistent with general mental health care standards. As research and practice continue to advance, however, therapeutic standards may change. Moreover, particular situations may require a particularized therapeutic response not addressed or included in this book. For these reasons and because human and mechanical errors sometimes occur, we recommend that readers follow the advice of psychologists or other therapists directly involved in their care or the care of a member of their family.

Unless otherwise indicated, all figures and images in the book are copyright Ken Tackett and used with permission.

Published by
APA LifeTools
750 First Street, NE
Washington, DC 20002
https://www.apa.org

Order Department
https://www.apa.org/pubs/books
order@apa.org

In the U.K., Europe, Africa, and the Middle East, copies may be ordered from Eurospan
https://www.eurospanbookstore.com/apa
info@eurospangroup.com

Typeset in Sabon by Circle Graphics, Inc., Reisterstown, MD

Printer: Gasch Printing, Odenton, MD
Cover Designer: Mark Karis

Library of Congress Cataloging-in-Publication Data

Names: Kendall-Tackett, Kathleen A., author.
Title: Breastfeeding doesn't need to suck : how to nurture your baby and
    your mental health / by Kathleen Kendall-Tackett.
Description: Washington, DC : American Psychological Association, [2022] |
    Includes bibliographical references and index.
Identifiers: LCCN 2021049623 (print) | LCCN 2021049624 (ebook) |
    ISBN 9781433833847 (paperback) | ISBN 9781433839979 (ebook)
Subjects: LCSH: Breastfeeding. | Breastfeeding--Psychological aspects. |
    BISAC: HEALTH & FITNESS / Breastfeeding | MEDICAL / Nursing /
    Maternity, Perinatal, Women's Health
Classification: LCC RJ216 .K425 2022 (print) | LCC RJ216 (ebook) |
    DDC 649/.33--dc23/eng/20211121
LC record available at https://lccn.loc.gov/2021049623
LC ebook record available at https://lccn.loc.gov/2021049624

https://doi.org/10.1037/0000287-000

Printed in the United States of America

10 9 8 7 6 5 4 3 2 1

CONTENTS

PREFACE

As a new mother, you're in the midst of the biggest transition of your life. You've been entrusted with a tiny, fragile human life, and decisions you make now can have long-range effects. If you're feeling a bit tearful, know that you are not alone. Most mothers face similar fears. Their heart's desire is to be good mothers, and they wonder if they will ever measure up. The last thing they need is problems breastfeeding.

If you've picked up this book, either breastfeeding is not working and you want to know why or you've heard the horror stories and are now scared to death. You feel that you "should" breastfeed because we all know "breast is best"; however, you're not sure if you're up for weeks of agony. I can't say I blame you.

In a perfect world, I'd love to see breastfeeding go well for all mothers right from the start, that they had support throughout their journeys, and that they reached their breastfeeding goals. However, this is the real world, and our lives rarely go according to plan. It's so different from how you imagined it. Here's what I want you to know: Breastfeeding can be challenging, especially in the beginning, but challenging is way different from impossible.

Where this book differs from others on the market is that I am focusing on *you*. If breastfeeding currently sucks, let's fix it. You should not have to suffer to feed your baby. I'm not going to talk much about why breastfeeding is good for your baby. There are tons of good books out there covering that topic (and you probably know that bit by heart). Instead, I am going to talk a lot about why breastfeeding is good for you.

Mothering rhetoric tends to gravitate to one of two positions with regard to caring for your baby. The first position is that everything is about the baby and that mothers should endure even weeks of severe pain. I've been at conferences where I've heard that if you're not responding to every baby sound, *you're damaging your baby's brain.* Wow, that's intense! It's also not true. It is especially important to answer your baby's cries because that's your baby's only way to communicate with you, but there is a bit of give in the system that can allow you to finish going to the bathroom. (Although few will say this publicly, there are many mothers who have nursed their babies while sitting on the toilet.)

At the other extreme, some advisors will make postpartum entirely about the mother. This approach promotes a lot of mother–baby separation and nonresponsive care. One mental health provider that I know uses cognitive therapy to teach mothers not to respond to their babies. That's not great either.

There is a third way: It is possible to take good care of yourself while caring for your baby. The fact is that your newborn is highly vulnerable and needs you. There will be a period of time when your baby's needs trump yours. However, that doesn't mean you should get lost in the process; your needs are important too.

We'll talk a lot about the importance of responsive care throughout this book. That means that when your baby cries, you come. It also means that when your baby wants to engage, you play (this is when the joy happens). However, this also means that you can safely put your baby on a blanket on the floor or in their car seat if you need to use the bathroom. It is possible to take good care of yourself while caring for your baby.

WHAT CAN MAKE BREASTFEEDING SUCK?

In the course of my travels, I've spoken with thousands of new mothers and the health care providers who work with them. Some things have definitely improved in terms of breastfeeding support, but there are still far too many mothers falling through the cracks. In the process of writing this book, I developed a brief survey that included 361 mothers from my Facebook page. It wasn't a formal study; I wanted to get a sense of the current breastfeeding landscape and what mothers were encountering. Most of these mothers had had successful breastfeeding experiences, which meant that they met their breastfeeding goals and breastfed for as long as they wanted. Yet the majority had experienced challenges in the first few weeks.

By far, the most common problem was painful latch, with 57% reporting this. Thirty-nine percent of mothers said that breast-feeding was exhausting, and another 39% worried about whether their babies were getting enough to eat. Thirty-five percent reported postpartum anxiety, and 23% had postpartum depression. Other common problems included a delay in their milk "coming in" (21%), low milk supply (22%), too much milk (23%), that they didn't know how to latch their baby (23%), 25% had to supplement, and 24% had a breast infection or yeast infection. Thirty-two percent had a baby with tongue-tie, 16% said their baby cried a lot, and 22% said their baby was not gaining well.

There is so much information out there. You may not know what to do next. As you look ahead, think of me as your gigantic bodyguard. My job is to walk you through the gauntlet of paparazzi shouting comments at you. Effective bodyguards shield their clients as they get them to safety. That is what I hope to do for you. With that in mind, here's I want for you:

- *To be pain-free.* Please don't listen to the voices who will tell you that pain is "normal." I know that many mothers experience it, but that makes it common, not normal. Pain is an important signal from your body. As my friend and breast-feeding medicine specialist Dr. Tina Smillie says, "If you have a rock in your shoe, you stop and take the rock out. You don't figure out how to walk with the rock."

    Unfortunately, mothers in pain think that pain means they are doing it "wrong." Many things can cause pain that have nothing to do with how you are doing it. For example, it could be an infection or something inside your baby's mouth. If you are experiencing pain, I want you to have the information you need to problem-solve or find the help you need.

- *To be confident.* I want you to know for sure that your baby is getting enough to eat—from you. If there is a problem, I want you to know how to spot it and what to do about it. You are amazing, and so is your body.

    As a new mother, you will receive a lot of advice, and when it comes to that, it's okay to listen to your gut. Lactation is largely a clinical field. Our evidence base is growing, but practice often precedes evidence. With different aspects of care, you'll find a lot of "true believers." If what they are telling you to do does not sit right with your gut, it doesn't matter how many people recommend it—you don't have to do it. Just because someone is adamant doesn't mean they are right, and "I tried it and it worked" is not evidence. What people recommend may help you too, but feel free to gather more information before you proceed, and then you may decide to ignore it altogether.

- *To feel in control.* So many things can happen in women's lives that are beyond our control. I've outlined some of the obstacles that you may run into in your breastfeeding journey. Unfortunately, obstacles are part of life. Can you overcome them? My response is a resounding *yes*. While breastfeeding is natural, it is also learned. If it's learned, then you and your baby can learn it.
- *To protect and support your mental health.* I don't want you struggling. I am a board-certified lactation consultant and a psychologist. You will never, ever hear from me "Just keep on breastfeeding, no matter what!" Mothers I've worked with over the years have run into that kind of advice, and it's so wrong. I don't want you in misery for weeks (or days). That's not good for anyone.

    Conversely, I don't agree with providers who will tell you to chuck breastfeeding as if it doesn't matter, without any attempt to fix the problem. If you choose to quit, that's your right, but so often, I hear stories of mothers being told to quit "to protect their mental health." I can't tell you the number of mothers I've spoken with who call me crying because they've just been diagnosed with postpartum depression and were told they need to quit breastfeeding. "And this is the only thing that is going well."

The decision to continue, or not, is yours alone.

I was recently at a conference and heard a speaker say that if a mother is at risk for not breastfeeding, she approaches her and says, "What can I do to help ensure that your baby has human milk?" The mother and her wishes and desires were totally taken out of the equation. That, in a nutshell, is what is wrong with much of the common breastfeeding advice. It's not about the mother at all; she is only the purveyor of the product. Don't get me wrong, your baby is super important, but your baby is only one half of the mother–baby couplet. You are a pair, and you're both important.

I'll walk you through the breastfeeding basics, but always looking at it through the lens of how breastfeeding affects you. I don't cover every topic, but where more information is needed, I'll refer you to other resources. I want to make sure that you have the basic tools you need to have a good breastfeeding experience. I'll also show you why, physiologically, breastfeeding protects your mental health and the things that might interfere with that protection.

Because of the focus of this book, I cover topics that other books on breastfeeding only touch on, such as postpartum anxiety, depression, and posttraumatic stress disorder. I discuss how your birth experience or previous traumatic events may be influencing your breastfeeding experience. I also cover sleep in some detail because it's one of the most salient issues for young families. You'll get a lot of bad advice about sleep, and I'd like to counter it with evidence. I also spend an entire section discussing social support; everyone says you need this, but they are often vague about what it is. Support can be tricky because it involves human relationships, and those by nature are often complicated. What looks like "support" to outsiders may not feel like support to you, and that's what matters. Finally, I describe what you can do if you cannot reach your breastfeeding goals. If that happens, all is not lost; there are many things you can still do.

You are investing time in mastering a difficult skill. Every bit you do is important for your baby, and it's also important for you. My goal is to walk you through this time. You deserve respect, to be cared for, and to be listened to—your opinion matters.

Don't worry so much about doing everything right. Life is messy, and you will make mistakes. But remember that you are your baby's favorite person. That's both an honor and a terrifying responsibility.

Let's begin.

ACKNOWLEDGMENTS

This book came to be in an unusual way. I had just been elected to the American Psychological Association's (APA's) Publications & Communications (P&C) Board, and it was my first meeting. We were introducing ourselves, and I said that I was a health psychologist and board-certified lactation consultant and could see a few eye rolls because I had admitted to being part of such a "girly" field. Emily Ekle, APA's acquisitions director, made a beeline for me at lunch and asked if I would like to write a book for them on breastfeeding. I knew all the folks at APA because I had written other books for them, edit one of their journals, and was now on P&C with them. Emily had a vision for what this book could be, and I appreciate the opportunity, even if she thinks I have crappy taste in beer. To sweeten the pot, I also got to work with my favorite editor at APA, Linda McCarter, who has enlivened up many a dull reception and shares my passion for Irish history and trying all the liquor a bored bartender offered us 1 tablespoon at a time. And although they didn't work directly on this project, I want to give a shout out to my great colleagues at APA Publishing: Jasper Simons, Annie Hill, Steph Pollock, Sheena Mouton, Anthony Oulette, and Rose Sokol, who make my jobs as journal editor and P&C Board member a joy.

I'd also like to thank Sarah Calabi, who was my developmental editor on this project, and the three anonymous reviewers. The four of them thoroughly reviewed my book and gave such thoughtful feedback. I know the book is better because of their hard work. Their many comments kept me busy and working late for weeks, but I'm so glad that I did. Thank you for all the care you poured into this manuscript.

My family has been intimately involved with this project from the beginning, especially my sons, Ken and Chris. They both work for me at my publishing company and used their skills to help me finish this book: Ken illustrated and Chris copyedited. My husband picked up the slack around the house and offered moral support and much-needed snacks when I was pressing toward my deadline (I'll work those off later). This book would not have been possible without their help.

My assistant, Jadine Sturgill, has held down the fort for months and made sure that I didn't miss important meetings or webinars that I was presenting at. I could not have finished without her help (or a lot of people would have been mad). Thank you, my friend.

Two other people have been pivotal to me completing this book: Kevin Jennings and Diane Sanford. Both talked me through mental blocks and Kevin helped me review my schedule to find time to write. Especially since we are in the midst of COVID, and my journal editing duties drastically increased, that was no mean feat. I appreciate you both.

I would also like to thank the 361 mothers who participated in our survey. You gave me real insight into the current birthing and breastfeeding landscape and told me what it was *really* like. Your stories added richness to this narrative. Thank you for sharing your stories with me.

I

THE FUNDAMENTALS

INTRODUCTION: THE FUNDAMENTALS

How you feed your baby is your first major parenting decision. As you step off the precipice into the unknown, it can be scary as hell. In some ways, the stakes could not be higher. Because of this, a surprising number of people want to manhandle your decision: your friends and family, your health care providers, and people who want to sell you things—from breastfeeding cookies, to pumps, to baby gear, to infant formula—all want to have a say.

Part I of this book describes a bit about the huge change in your life. I refer to these principles throughout the rest of the book, but if you are having a specific concern, please skip ahead to the sections that seem most relevant. You can always come back to this section. I hope these chapters reassure you and let you know that what you are experiencing is normal. Postpartum is intense and relatively short, but it doesn't feel that way when you're going through it.

Congratulations, Mom! It's going to be okay.

CHAPTER 1

A PRIMER ON BREASTFEEDING

Before I move into the particulars of breastfeeding, I thought a few ground rules might be helpful to frame our discussion.

HOW YOU FEED YOUR BABY IS YOUR BUSINESS—PERIOD

Infant feeding is one of those topics that enlivens everyone's passions. Parenting involves many decisions over your child's life, and you will frequently find that there are distinct camps on many issues, but none seems to inspire vehemence as much as feeding.

So much of the conversation around breastfeeding is unkind and, frankly, awful. For many new mothers, social media becomes a lifeline of support, but it can also be a sewer of misinformation and—dare I say it?—hate. Learning to deflect is an important parenting skill. "This is what works best for our family" is one of the handiest sentences that you can learn.

Some of this unhelpful rhetoric started off with good intentions (you know what they say about those, right?). We learned that when the lactation field said "breast is best," mothers interpreted that as "breastfeeding is nice if you can do it." Instead, we wanted mothers to realize that breastfeeding is the biological norm, so we adopted "risk-based" language to let you know what would happen if breastfeeding was not happening (e.g., "formula increases the risk of death and disease by X times"). As you can imagine, mothers hated that language. I knew so many mothers who genuinely suffered and had no decent support, and the risk-based language was salt in the wound.

A SECURE ATTACHMENT SUPERSEDES BREASTFEEDING AS A PARENTING GOAL

That's probably a strange statement to see in a breastfeeding book, but it's true. Although I am a health psychologist, my training is in developmental psychology. I've often joked that my PhD was useless to me as a new mother. In retrospect, I know that's not entirely true. One thing it gave me was confidence in babies' innate drive to grow and develop. You don't need to hover over every little thing; just interact with and love them, and they will grow.

The most important goal in early parenting is fostering a secure attachment with your baby, and you do that with responsive care. Do you want a smart baby? A baby who does well in school and gets along with their peers? Do you want a baby who is resilient and healthy as an adult? A secure attachment does all of that (Owenz, 2021; Schore, 2001).

Breastfeeding facilitates a secure attachment because you have to respond to your baby to make it work, but you may be surprised to learn that you don't have to breastfeed to have a secure attachment. We know this because most of the early research on attachment was done with formula-feeding infants.

You may think I'm saying that breastfeeding doesn't matter. Of course, it does, but there's even a bigger prize at stake. If you have encountered breastfeeding difficulties, all is not lost. The big prize—secure attachment—is still quite attainable.

BREASTFEEDING IS MORE THAN MILK

Unfortunately, many breastfeeding campaigns have focused entirely on milk, which reflects the influence of the bottle-feeding culture. When we say human milk is a better "product" than formula, we miss the boat. Human milk is the ideal food for babies. It's not just better ingredients; it's living tissue that includes active white blood cells to fight infection. You do lose some of these cells when you freeze milk, but even then, it still protects your baby. Something cooked up in a lab will never do that. Campaigns that focus only on providing milk miss something crucial: Breastfeeding is also a relationship. In other words, breastfeeding is more than milk.

What happens if a mother is not fully able to feed her baby at the breast? Is there anything she can do? Yes! Please keep reading. Even if mothers cannot fully breastfeed, they can still feed in such a way as to foster a secure attachment.

RULE NUMBER 1: FEED THE BABY

People sometimes slander breastfeeding supporters, saying that we impose our agenda on mothers, even when babies' weights are faltering or there are obvious signs of problems. When you hear a tragic story, there's often a provider who missed important cues and did not do a proper evaluation.

If a mother thinks something is wrong, if the baby is distressed or not gaining weight, we always need to evaluate the mother and baby. It could be that everything is okay, and we can reassure the mother. If there is a problem, however, supplementation may be necessary; that does not mean the end of breastfeeding. In most cases, supplementation is temporary and a bridge to overcoming a problem.

In the past, supplementation has gotten a bad rap because it was overused. You will still find health care providers who suggest supplementing rather than addressing a breastfeeding problem or referring mothers to someone who can help. Skilled lactation support is critical, and our goal is to address problems as quickly as possible while ensuring that the baby has enough to eat.

SOME CHALLENGES OF EARLY MOTHERHOOD ARE NOT RELATED TO BREASTFEEDING

Having a baby is one of the biggest things you will ever do. The changes it creates in your life are seismic. Unfortunately, our culture responds with a resounding "Meh!" When you're in the midst of it, it's easy to think that all the challenges you face in the early weeks are because of breastfeeding. Then the siren song of the formula companies says, "It would be so much easier if you just gave this up." Unfortunately, many mothers have found that giving up breastfeeding didn't help as much as they hoped and may have introduced some new challenges.

You may have had some impossible expectations for how easy this will be because you see those images everywhere. The new mother is perfectly turned out, in a well-appointed home, next to her doting partner. That's not your reality. You chance a quick look in the mirror, and you see a bleary-eyed specter staring back at you in a faded T-shirt with a splatter of baby spit-up on your shoulder. Your BC (before children) friends shrink back in horror as you answer the door. Fortunately, your friends with children know this is normal. Even better, this stage is temporary.

BREASTFEEDING CAN BE A LOT MORE WORK AT THE BEGINNING

Learning to breastfeed is an investment, but once you master it, it's a lot less work. You may be asking yourself, "Is it worth it?" This is what some of the mothers in my survey said:

> Be patient. Both you and the baby are new to this and learning from each other.

> It takes a few weeks in the beginning and gets easier.

> Trust your gut; it's hard work.

Kelly, a mother of a 3-week-old, told me this:

> You hear about all the problems with breastfeeding, but what they don't tell you is how nice it is. It's like you're in your own little love bubble.

A mother shared that she went into breastfeeding with some trepidation and encountered a number of problems because her babies had health problems. She had this to say:

> Before having my first baby, I witnessed a few of my friends having difficulty with breastfeeding. There were a variety of issues, but I did see how their struggle affected them personally. They expressed how frustrating it was and the sense of failure they felt. I did not come from a background of breastfeeders. It was not something I felt super strongly about, but knew I would like to try it and see how it went. . . . Overall, I had wonderful experiences with breastfeeding and would have loved to have been able to do it longer. . . . *I never would have thought I would have been someone to try to persuade a new mama to really put their trust in the benefits of breastfeeding, but I definitely am. There is no connection like it.* (emphasis added)

Another mother shared this story. She had a difficult birth and did not receive good breastfeeding support. After having struggled and gone through so much, she had this to say:

> I had planned a homebirth. Had a long prodromal labor that lasted 5 days. Got to 8 cm and then midwife realized baby was breech and I transferred to hospital where I had a cesarean. I felt overwhelmed, frightened, and had very little support from midwife and hospital staff. My son was admitted to the NICU for 24 hours, and they pushed formula supplementation. Breast-feeding was extremely painful, but the IBCLC [International Board Certified Lactation Consultant] at hospital kept saying, "Looks great, keep doing the same thing!" I saw three different IBCLCs after discharge and my baby diagnosed with tongue-tie, but the frenotomy didn't work well. Breastfeeding was painful for first 4 months, and I struggled with supply due to bad latch. It finally clicked after 4 months and can't think of anything in my life I am prouder of than making that work!

I don't want you to struggle for weeks or months, but I'm struck by what she said in the end. When it finally worked, she was so proud of what she had done. I'd like to close this chapter with these lovely words by a longtime lactation consultant, Chris Auer. It lines up beautifully with the message of this chapter:

> I have been captivated by watching the Netflix series *Babies*. The breastfeeding relationship is so beautifully portrayed. What a gift you have been given to witness breastfeeding couplet interactions. We see a mom relax into the moment once her baby latches. Because her well-being is so critical to the baby's well-being, nurturing the mother and helping her assume her maternal role, even when the latch isn't achieved, is crucial. Beyond that, the series records skin-to-skin contact interactions. It's a gentle reminder to promote this among the adopting parents and those who opt not to breastfeed. It's the rare mother who hasn't imprinted the first contact with her newborn. She remembers. The mirroring goes both ways.

CHAPTER 2

THE FIVE I's OF NEW MOTHERHOOD

The early days of motherhood are a jolt to the system. You may attribute your sense of overwhelm to breastfeeding, but some of the challenges you face are more likely simply due to being a new mother. It's just so different, and in your right-brain state, you may feel that it will be this way forever. Formula seems like the way out: "Maybe it's possible to have a bit of my old life back again." Unfortunately, if you stop breastfeeding, the problems may continue because these challenges are inherent to postpartum no matter how you feed your baby. As Psychologist Dr. Amy Brown (2019) noted, "Mothering is the most powerful of all biological capacities and among the most disempowering of social experiences" (p. 148).

THE "FIVE I's" OF NEW MOTHERHOOD: WHY THE FIRST FEW WEEKS CAN BE A BEAR

I've summarized some of the common challenges of the early weeks as "the Five I's of new motherhood." If you recognize these challenges, they will be easier to cope with. Unabated, they prey on your mind and make you believe that breastfeeding is impossible.

Idleness

Western culture values productivity and busyness: "If you're not busy, you're not living up to your potential, contributing to society, or earning your keep." You might read "idleness" and think "Are you kidding me? I'm super busy." If that's you, skip ahead to the next section. However, in the early days, many new mothers are challenged with the reality of spending their days sitting, holding the baby, and nursing the baby. In the meantime, life is going on. You feel you should be doing things around the house, or for work, or something. Gone are the days of your to-do lists, the business appointments, the time when you got to the end of the day and had something to show for it. What happened to your life? Actor Brooke Shields (2005) said this:

> I love schedules but prefer to be the person making them. It occurred to me that my life was no longer my own and that I was a prisoner to a small, squeaking creature. I did not like it one bit. I felt stuck. I did not want the responsibility this situation demanded. (p. 70)

To cope with idleness, some reframing might help. Think about the body's brilliant design. You've just had a baby and need time to recover. Your baby needs time to adjust to the world. Doesn't it make perfect sense that your body is simply hitting the pause button on your life? It's saying, "just be for a moment." Soon you will be quite busy again, but take a breath and let your body heal.

Others may reinforce the idea that you need to be "productive." They'll make snide remarks like "I didn't need to take any time off. My work is important. I wasn't weak. I exercised during pregnancy." Blah, blah, blah. This is so ingrained in our culture—it's like air; we don't even notice it.

This time is not idle (although it may feel like it). You're establishing critical neural pathways for you and your baby to establish your milk production. You are the duck on the pond; from the outside, it may look like you're doing nothing, but under the water, there's loads of activity. What you are craving is some structure. I'll offer some practical guidance. You can feel better about this time. This is (fortunately) brief, and what you are doing is so important. Postpartum doula Salle Webber (2012) described it like this:

> When a woman gives birth for the first time, she is forever transformed; the uninitiated young female metamorphoses into full womanhood. She has been entrusted with a baby, and the urging of her body continues to keep her focused on her new role. Being in constant service to a newborn is unlike any other job she has had, but after nine months of pregnancy, labor, and delivery, a woman's body and psyche are attuned to this new life. (p. 9)

Isolation

In his book *Bowling Alone*, Dr. Robert Putnam (2000) described how isolated Americans have become over the past generation, to the point where bowling leagues (and other social groups) have vanished and we're more likely to go bowling alone. Postpartum seems to exacerbate this effect. We have historical precedent for understanding the effects of social isolation. Once upon a time, frontier women lived in little cabins, and men would vanish for weeks at a time in search of game, to trap, or to herd cattle. Women were alone with small children and no other adults. "Cabin fever" is a real thing; women went crazy from the social isolation of it all.

Dr. Glenda Matthews (1987) wrote a great social history of domesticity in the United States called *"Just a Housewife": The Rise and Fall of Domesticity in America*. She described how women in the 1950s were often so isolated in the newly created suburbs that they would listen to the radio to hear another human voice during the day. They were in neighborhoods with no car and no place to walk to. They were starved for adult companionship.

A new mother called me several times during a particularly brutal winter in northern New England. We had tons of snow that year, and she was trapped in her house all day with two small children; she was slowly going mad. I urged her to get the kids into their snowsuits, get in the car, and go someplace—any place, even the drive-thru at McDonald's. She needed to interact with other people.

Isolation can hit like a hammer, especially once your partner goes back to work or your support person goes home. Another mother told me that when she was home with a new baby, her husband was a medical resident, which meant working 80 to 100 hours a week. They'd moved, and she didn't know anyone, and it was winter in a place with a lot of snow. Once the snow melted, she finally got to meet people, and her depression got better. She was surprised that she had gotten depressed in this situation. I told her that I would have been surprised if she hadn't, given the number of stressors she endured.

Salle Webber (2012) also described the effects of isolation and the abrupt change from being constantly "busy" to stopping to care for a new baby:

> While friends and family are thrilled about the new baby, they are very busy with their own lives. The new mom may find herself spending hours at a time alone at home with her newborn. She may be coming from a fast-paced job with lots of stimulation, or a full social life, and now spends hours walking the floor hoping to put the baby to sleep, often in her pajamas all day, forgetting when she last brushed her teeth. It is vital to retain perspective at this time, to know this is temporary and precious. Postpartum depression threatens as a mom may begin to feel her own needs unmet. She requires compassion and humor, and small breaks from her responsibilities. (pp. 37–38)

If you see other people, especially friends or coworkers who do not have children, you may feel isolated because you are now so different from them. Even when all goes well, birth is a radical and transformative event. You may find it hard to express that—and the massive changes you've been through—to people who haven't experienced it themselves. It's not unlike a combat vet returning from a war zone.

If you wonder why this isolation is bothering you, know this: Social isolation is a form of torture. In prisons, solitary confinement is considered "cruel and unusual." Are you tougher than a prisoner? Why would you think that you would not be affected by this?

Incompetence

Another challenge of early mothering is incompetence. Before you had your baby, you were probably good at things. You had a job that used your brain; you knew how to solve problems and get through your day. Then you had this little being, and suddenly everything is new—and you're good at none of it. Some mothers find these feelings so intolerable that they rush back to work, even before the end of their maternity leaves. They want to be back to a place where they know how to do things. I've observed that older mothers often find this harder than younger ones because they've been independent longer, but it is hard for everyone.

Let's reframe this one too. You're not incompetent—you're learning; there's a big difference. You're also using a part of your brain that may not have had much exercise in our left-brain world. (How do you feel when you use a new muscle for the first time?) In a few short weeks, you will emerge from this time and be awed at how much you've learned. When you're in the right-brain state, it seems this will last forever. It doesn't, but here's something for your left-brain to hang on to. Grab a calendar and mark off 40 days from now. I guarantee that you will look back and be amazed at the ubercompetence you've acquired.

Identity

Before children, you were your own person. You had things you enjoyed and were proud of. If you have a partner, that is one type of identity, but you're still a separate adult. Now you're a mother. You may have wanted it (longed for it, even), and you wouldn't go back, but some people seem to be a little less interested in what you have to say. If you are home with a new baby, your day is full of breastfeeding, poopy diapers, and keeping your head above water. Your scope has narrowed as you focus on this one thing.

There are a couple of things to mention here. First, this stage is temporary. I've said that before, but it bears repeating. Second, yes, your identity has changed, but you're still you, and your brain is still there. The old you hasn't gone away; you've added a new dimension. You've created a new life, and you are sustaining it with your body. That's an amazing and wondrous thing to be immensely proud of.

Intensity

The final I is intensity. If you're not prepared for it, it can knock you sideways. Mothering is relentless, and this new little being needs you all the time. You may feel like running away. Don't feel bad if you're not "loving every minute" or if you feel touched out by the end of the day. That's pretty normal.

For many mothers, this time feels super intense because they need to hold their babies so much. They wonder if it will be forever. It won't be. Dr. Suzanne Colson (2019) described postpartum as helping your baby transition "from Womb to World." What feels like intensity to you is part of the transition for your baby. Mothers often asked Colson, a former midwife in the United Kingdom, how long they should hold their babies. Colson told mothers to hold their babies as much as they liked but reminded them that before birth, their babies were held 24/7, so it's natural that they want to be held now. They like to smell their mother and hear her heartbeat; it's all they know.

It makes it worse when people tell you that you're holding your baby "too much." That can exacerbate your worries. This is just another example of poor advice that new mothers often receive. I hope I can alleviate your worries by telling you that there's no such thing as holding your baby too much. Do it for as long as you like.

Sometimes people will try to help you manage this intense time by swooping in and taking over baby care. Honestly, sometimes an extra pair of hands is good. You can take a shower, put on some fresh clothes, and possibly relax on your bed, but a couple of cautions are in order. First, if your baby gets passed around among too many people, they will be much fussier by the end of the day. Even newborns are aware of their surroundings, and too many handlers can lead to crying. Second, as a breastfeeding mother, you are establishing your milk production in those first few weeks. Although a short break can be great, longer breaks lead to missed feedings, which can lower milk production or increase your risk of mastitis. I'd suggest limiting your break times to 30 to 60 minutes at a time, picking up your baby if they start to cry.

Right now, breastfeeding is super intense because you are establishing your supply and your baby needs to be held all the time. Within a few short weeks, your investment will pay off. Your baby has a huge jump in brain development at 6 weeks. They still need to be held and fed, but things start feeling easier. Breastfeeding will be established, and it will seem a bit more regular. It's still subject to change, but the changes will feel easier to manage.

Right-brain thinking causes your sense of time to be distorted (see Chapter 3). Your mind spins with thoughts like "I can't stay like this forever. I need to have a life. I have to get back to normal," so you plot your getaway. Sometimes your desire for a bit of space is intense. You want it, you *need* it, and you feel that you just can't cope.

If you're there now, remember this: If you need a bit of space, you can take it. Feed your baby first, and figure you've got about an hour. Perhaps you can take your baby along someplace else. Sometimes just being in a different space can help.

To reiterate what I said earlier, this phase is temporary. Get your calendar and count 40 days from when you gave birth. You'll be a mother from now on, but you won't always be a new mother, and that makes all the difference.

COPING STRATEGIES FOR THE FIVE I's

As you face the early weeks, the goal is to settle your mind while mastering breastfeeding and recuperating from birth. To help you with this time, here are some suggestions other mothers have shared and things I have tried myself. I recommend trying these ideas to see if they work for you and ignoring the rest.

Get Dressed Every Day

During the early days of COVID-19, many workers were sent home to work for the first time. While I enjoy telecommuting and have done it for many years, others were upset that they had to do it. One of my associates struggled quite a bit, so I shared some strategies I've learned through trial and error.

The first thing I suggested is to get dressed every day. It sounds simple, but it makes a difference in your outlook. Although you can spend the entire day in your pajamas, it may make you feel "sick." If you put on some clean clothes, you will feel better. Ask whoever helps you to keep up with the laundry so that you always have clean clothes available. You don't need to dress for the office, but a clean T-shirt and yoga pants will cheer you and structure your day by marking day versus night.

Avoid Long Periods of Silence

Sometimes silence is a gift, but if you are home alone all day, silence can increase your feelings of isolation. While I don't necessarily like the TV blaring all day, I understand the impulse to leave it on. I'm not recommending that, but to break the silence, you can listen to music. You can go outside and walk around. You can go to a park or coffee shop, just to be around other people. If you are having trouble being alone with your thoughts, especially if you are ruminating, break it up and give your brain something else to chew on. It will really help.

If you are feeling cut off from the outside world, you could listen to some podcasts. You may feel so sleep-deprived that you have a hard time following it. If that's the case, so what? You'll get the gist of it and that may be enough to help you feel connected to the world, and it will break up the silence. Your concentration will come back. It's just in a different place right now.

Get a Baby Sling

If you feel like all you can do is sit on a couch, a sling will help. Slings are comfortable and babies generally love them. I'm not a big fan of tons of gear, but this piece is super helpful. In terms of this chapter, a sling will also make it easier to get up and do things. If you want to make yourself a snack or do a couple of dishes (and I hope you don't have to do all of that, but you might want to), you have at least one hand free. You may need at least one hand on your baby, but you can move around.

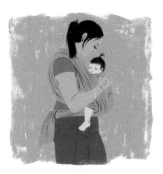

A baby sling can make it quite a bit easier to move about during the day.

Get a Rolling Table

This is a handy object that I discovered after shoulder surgery when I was also one-handed for weeks. Although I couldn't type emails with only one hand, I could at least use my computer. They can also be a place to hold your phone, water bottle, and snacks and are inexpensive to rent from medical supply companies.

Have a Loose Schedule

Although nursing will be unpredictable in the beginning, having a loose schedule can help your mental well-being. What time will you have lunch? When will you take a nap? When will you go outside?

One-Handed Tasks

If you would feel better doing "something," set up a few tasks that you can do one-handed, such as reviewing your bills or going through your mail. Having a few small tasks can break up your day and remind you of the life you will have again.

Read Something You Enjoy

This is not the time to finally read *War and Peace*, but is there something fun, frivolous, and entertaining you'd enjoy? Order yourself a stack of books or magazines or head to your local library.

Limit Phone Time

I know your phone may seem like a lifeline, but I'd strongly suggest limiting your phone time to no more than 2 hours per day. When you are glued to your phone, you disengage from your baby, and to your baby, it seems like you are depressed. This stresses babies and raises their cortisol levels. Use a timer or an app that shuts down your phone time after a couple of hours.

Get Outside Most Days

Even if you don't drive someplace, just walking outside for a few minutes can lift your spirits. If you're starting to feel trapped in the house, step outside. If you're up to it, you can take a walk with your baby. The fresh air will be good for both of you.

Keep the Area Where You Spend Most of Your Time Tidy

While I don't think you should be doing housework, you may feel better if the space where you are spending the most time is picked up. As far as I'm concerned, the rest of the house can look like a bomb went off, but a small pocket of order will be good for your mental state.

CONCLUSION

The postpartum period is relatively short, but it doesn't feel that way when you're in the midst of it. Once you realize that many mothers find this time challenging, you can stop expecting yourself to be happy all the time. In your mind, try to separate the difficulties of postpartum from any breastfeeding challenges you may be encountering. Sometimes mothers attribute the challenges that they are facing to breastfeeding and stop, only to find that the problems are still there. You're doing something amazing, even if you don't feel "productive." Honestly, what's more productive than making and feeding another human being? It helps to keep some perspective. Be kind to yourself—know that this too shall pass.

CHAPTER 3

BREASTFEEDING: LEARNED OR INSTINCTUAL?

Many mothers who struggle with breastfeeding wonder why they can't do it. Many have been told that breastfeeding is "natural" and both they and their baby will know how to do it. That advice might give you confidence to trust the process. Or, if you're struggling, you may think that you don't have "maternal instincts." How are you supposed to be a mother without those?

Some mothers in my survey said that "breastfeeding is natural" was among the worst advice that they received. (To be fair, an equal number said it was the most helpful advice.) At the very least, I hope you can see that not everyone finds that advice to be helpful, and in some circumstances, it can make you feel worse. Dr. Amy Brown (2019) described this well:

> Breastfeeding might be natural and normal and all these words, but that doesn't make it easy. Just as it often takes time to develop any physical skill . . ., it can take time to get the hang of breastfeeding. It might look as straightforward as just latching that baby on the breast, but a whole load of factors are often against us, from a stressful birth to being in an uncomfortable position through to barely having seen anyone else breastfeed so we are less instinctively aware of how to hold and position the baby. (p. 110)

A BRIEF HISTORY OF BREASTFEEDING ADVICE

Throughout much of human history, women breastfed or hired (or forced) someone else to do it. In cultures in which babies weren't breastfed, the infant mortality rate was shockingly high. Until fairly recently in human history, there was no safe alternative. In the modern era, breastfeeding came close to extinction in the developed world. Proponents of so-called scientific mothering in the 1920s and 1930s told mothers that formula (named as such because of its "scientific" origins) was better for babies than their own milk.

By the 1950s and 1960s, breastfeeding rates hit rock bottom, and it almost died out, but a small percentage of intrepid mothers still wanted to breastfeed, with no support and pretty much everything against them. Breastfeeding researchers at this time believed that breastfeeding is a 100% learned behavior. If mothers were going to do it, they had to be directly taught. So professionals started teaching mothers and adopted pretty rigid ways of teaching, with a particular focus on the baby's position. Some mothers were able to adapt to this and go on to have successful breastfeeding experiences. Unfortunately, many others did not, partly because what was taught often created problems, such as sore nipples (Colson, 2019). In addition, many of the teachers learned different things and passed them along to mothers.

Hospitals sometimes compounded the problem. Your day nurse says one thing, the night nurse another, and the lactation consultant yet another. Mothers get so confused. British lactation consultant Lucy Ruddle, author of *Relactation* (2020) and *Mixed-Up* (2021), recently posted what follows on her Facebook page. I thought it was a fabulous illustration of what it's like for new mothers to receive this torrent of conflicting information: super confusing and frustrating. The tone is deliberately sarcastic for that reason. Judging by the number of shares, I think it resonated with many mothers' experiences. I asked her permission to share it.

> Idk why y'all struggle so much. Breastfeeding is easy. All you have to do is . . .

1. Pick up on early hunger cues.
   a. But if you're too early, you'll need to change their nappy and remove their clothes to wake them up.
   b. And if you happen to miss a cue because you were attending to your own basic needs, you'll have to calm the baby before latching them.
2. Remember nose to nipple, tummy to mummy, and head free to tip back. Unless your nipples point any direction other than straight out and unless your boobs are large, small, floppy, or a bit wonky.
   a. Tummy to mummy never works
   b. But have you tried tummy to mummy?
3. Never touch your breast. Unless your baby needs help latching.
   a. But not like that
   b. And don't do "that" too long either
   c. MASTITIS
4. Don't time or limit feeds.
   a. Unless your baby isn't gaining weight
   b. But also don't restrict breast access for slow-weight-gain babies
   c. Unless you should
5. Feed them every 3 hours
   a. Unless they want feeding every 2 hours
   b. But every hour is too much
   c. Unless it's not too much
6. If breastfeeding hurts, get support.
   a. Except if your pain is described as normal
   b. Breastfeeding shouldn't hurt
   c. But sometimes it hurts

7. Don't use a nipple shield.
   a. Unless you need one
   b. But do you REALLY need one?
   c. Hmm . . .
8. Pumping in the first 6 weeks is terrible.
   a. Except when it's needed
9. Don't use cross cradle.
   a. Why aren't you using cross cradle?
   b. No, not like that
10. Formula is terrible.
    a. Formula is brilliant
    b. Just feel guilty, ok?

See, easy! (Used with permission)

THE PARADIGM SHIFT

Then something magical happened. We learned that human babies could crawl to the breast like other mammals and attach to it. No one thought they could do that until Righard and Alade (1990) showed that they could. UNICEF India released a remarkable video, *Breast Crawl*, that has had almost a million views on YouTube showing a baby crawling and attaching to her mother's breast.

The UNICEF India video shows that babies are competent when it comes to getting on the breast.

The *Breast Crawl* video shows you what an amazing and complex system the mother–baby unit is. So, why have most professionals never seen this? That's simple; it's because hospital routines interfere with it. In that first hour after birth, hospital staff often whisk the baby away to clean, check, and weigh them. That's starting to change, fortunately, but it is still standard practice at many institutions. When the professionals take the baby away, they remove the stimuli that release inborn behaviors. Babies need skin-to-skin contact with their mothers and time for these mechanisms to be released (Matthiesen et al., 2001). Several physicians who have seen the breast crawl with their patients told me that it takes about an hour for this to occur. Many practitioners are not patient enough to wait, and, in fairness, many did not realize that there is something they should wait for.

Once we learned that babies had instincts, many in the field started to wonder whether mothers did too. Into this conversation came Dr. Suzanne Colson, a midwife, and researcher from the United Kingdom. She argued that teaching mothers to breastfeed using "positioning and attachment" was counterproductive. She believed that mothers did indeed have instincts and that professionals were suppressing them (Colson, 2019). What Dr. Colson observed is that when mothers have quiet time with their babies, with the baby's cheek on the mother's breast, mothers stroke and touch their babies in a way that no one ever taught them to do. The same pattern appears in mother after mother in Colson's study, but the conditions have to be right to see this.

IT DOESN'T HAVE TO BE EITHER–OR. IT'S BOTH

Returning to our original question, do mothers need to be taught to breastfeed? I believe that breastfeeding is both instinctual and learned. It is a complex set of behaviors. "Instinctual" does not mean that I hand you a baby and you know just what to do. Instinctual means that under the right circumstances, with the right releasing stimuli, you will act in concert with your baby, doing things that no one taught you to do.

Unfortunately, we can suppress a mother's instincts to the point where it seems they don't exist and teach breastfeeding in some unhelpful ways. For example, I spoke with a new mother recently who took a 3-hour prenatal breastfeeding class. She came home and cried because it was so complicated. Instead of feeling empowering, she was overwhelmed with information and doubted she could do it. After 1 week of breastfeeding, she was miserable, with cracked and bleeding nipples, and ready to quit. We got on Zoom, I showed her a position, and within a couple of minutes, she was feeding *with no pain*. She asked why no one in her 3-hour class had shown her this position. Why indeed? I discuss this more in Chapter 5.

HOW WE LEARN MAKES A DIFFERENCE: RIGHT- VERSUS LEFT-BRAIN LEARNING

If breastfeeding is both learned and instinctual, then some teaching is necessary. However, judging from the number of women who experience problems, I think it's safe to say that the rigid models we have used in the past are not effective. Dr. Tina Smillie has often proposed a framework that I've found to be helpful in understanding how mothers learn to breastfeed: right- versus left-brain learning.

Decades ago, neuroscientists discovered that our cerebral cortex is divided into two sections that are connected by a thick bundle of nerves called the corpus callosum. In your day-to-day life, you use both parts of your brain all the time, but for certain activities, one side may dominate. For example, your language skills are mostly in your left side, and many believe that your creative skills are mostly on your right side.

Neuroscience has advanced a great deal since these initial distinctions were made, so the models are much more sophisticated than what I am presenting in this chapter. However, these constructs about left versus right brain have migrated to other fields, including business, education, and the arts, where they are useful for

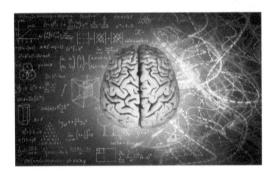

The two sides of your cerebral cortex do different things. Day to day, you use both sides, but for certain tasks, one side (or the other) predominates. Triff/Shutterstock.com.

understanding how people learn and function. What I'm describing is basically the more "general audience" version of this construct. This model tells us a lot about different ways of learning—for example, memorizing facts versus learning by doing. The functions of each side are described next.

Your Left Brain

Your left brain is amazing and is probably the side that has predominated for most of your adult life. It's the side of your brain that is

- logical
- verbal
- practical
- sequential (you think of things step-by-step)
- analytical
- objective

- focused on parts
- detail oriented

Your Right Brain

Your right brain is also amazing, and it's the side that many people find to be a lot more fun. Your right brain is

- emotional
- intuitive
- creative
- capable of synthesizing information
- subjective
- focused on wholes
- "big-picture" oriented
- attuned to symbols and images

The right brain also helps us form attachments. UCLA psychiatrist Dr. Allan Schore's (2000, 2001, 2009) seminal work described how all human attachment is based in the right brain. Given this, Schore (2000, 2009) has argued that mothers are wired to make right-brain to right-brain connections with their babies in the first few days of life.

When you're a new mother, you may believe that your brain no longer functions. Sleep deprivation certainly has a hand here, but feeling like your brain is fuzzy may also be a function of the right brain. Your brain is actually working quite well, but in a different way. Your left brain may temporarily be in the backseat, but it is still there and has never left.

To give you an idea about how this works, compare how you processed the lists about right and left brain versus how you processed the picture on page 29. You probably processed the picture instantly and immediately grasped the concept. Using your left brain, you reviewed the information sequentially when you went down the list.

As a writer and publisher, I work in a creative field and manage a whole team of creatives. Not surprisingly, I spend a lot of time using my right brain. It's a fun place to be, but when I'm working, I often lose track of time and may forget about appointments. My assistant, Jadine, acts like my left brain for me when I need to do creative work. To move my business forward, I need time to be right-brained, but I can't miss appointments or deadlines, so Jadine keeps track. In the same way, your partner or support person can assist you greatly if they keep track of left-brained stuff, such as appointments or writing down instructions.

There are many examples of right-brain learning, such as body memory. We learn to ride a bike with our bodies; you couldn't learn to do it through step-by-step instruction. Dancing is something where we start with our left brain (step, kick, slide) and then shift to our right brain. Once the steps become more of a body memory, we're not thinking about steps, and it's more fun. I think this is one reason why lactation consultants often want to reach over and adjust babies at the breast, even though it's no longer considered best practice; in some ways, it's easier to show (right brain) than to tell (left brain).

Applying This to Breastfeeding

According to Schore (2001, 2009), your right brain predominates postpartum to help you attach to your baby. Conveniently, breastfeeding is also a right-brained task. We absorb knowing how to do it by seeing breastfeeding mothers or breastfeeding images. That's one reason modern mothers may have trouble doing it—because they've rarely seen it. When we do see it, we remember it with our bodies more than our heads. It's much harder to do when you have to think it through step-by-step.

Another difficulty is the way we like to teach it. Although breastfeeding is a right-brain activity, we often teach it to your left brain. We load up mothers with tons of information and terminology, teaching it like it's a college course. The mother experiences it as "learn to breastfeed in 467 easy steps." We encourage them to use apps to keep track of minutes per side, the time between feedings, the time they slept. We've got them focused on the left-brain weeds instead of encouraging them to rest and spend time holding and hanging out with their babies.

CONCLUSION

The purpose of this chapter was to set up the framework for chapters that follow. I also wanted to reassure you if you are worried that you don't have "maternal instincts." You absolutely do. But bad advice may be suppressing them.

Breastfeeding is primarily a relationship, not a process. It is touch and contact and smell and looking into your baby's eyes. It is using your body to comfort your little one. You are the most important person in the world to your baby, and no one is better suited to the task. You're the one for this job. One mother said that this was the best advice she received:

> To do what worked for us. That it didn't have to be pretty, and I didn't have to have the best position. If the baby was happy and fed, then keep doing what I was doing.

As I'll describe in subsequent chapters, the "right" position is the one that works. If your baby is drinking well and you're not in pain, it's working. Once that's sorted, you can relax and enjoy your baby and not have to worry about anyone else's definition of "right."

CHAPTER 4

BREASTFEEDING AND YOUR MENTAL HEALTH

When mothers are struggling, mental health professionals can be quick to urge them to cut back on breastfeeding or to completely wean. I learned this by talking with mothers. Early in my career, I got many calls from depressed breastfeeding mothers from all over the United States. (I later found out that La Leche League International was giving out my home telephone number to all mothers who called their national hotline and said they were depressed.) They told me the same story: They had just been diagnosed with postpartum depression and were told to wean. Many mothers also said, "And this is the only thing that is going well for me."

I heard this story so many times, I was determined to find answers for them. In some cases, the mental health professional assumed that breastfeeding was too hard for them, even when it was going well. Others seemed to think that breastfeeding was largely disposable, especially "if the mother's mental health was at stake." I recently heard this from a psychologist who works with new mothers: "I will do whatever it takes to protect a mother's mental health. If she needs to stop breastfeeding, so be it."

Some professionals worry about transfer of medication into the mother's milk. When I first started doing this work, we had no resources that could help mothers looking for information. We didn't know if it was safe to breastfeed on antidepressants. We didn't know if it was wise to encourage them to continue. Fortunately, we now have many great resources, and I can tell you definitively that almost all antidepressants are compatible with breastfeeding. There is only one class of antidepressants that are not compatible with breastfeeding—the monoamine oxidase inhibitors (MAOIs)—and these are rarely prescribed.

I considered it progress when mental health providers at least tolerated breastfeeding, even if they couldn't actively support it. The next stage in thinking about mental health and breastfeeding came from an unlikely place: the field of psychoneuroimmunology (PNI). PNI researchers usually do not study breastfeeding, but Dr. Maureen Groer did (Groer & Davis, 2006; Groer & Kendall-Tackett, 2011). She found that the physical act of breastfeeding turned off the mother's inflammation response, which is key to understanding why breastfeeding protects maternal mental health. I was finally able to connect the dots after being invited to speak at a couple of conferences in 2006.

BREASTFEEDING CHANGES THE PHYSIOLOGY OF DEPRESSION

During that summer, I was asked to speak at the International Lactation Consultant Association conference on new developments in postpartum depression. At the same time, I was asked to present at a think-tank meeting at the University of Kentucky on the effects of violence against women and the risk of heart disease and diabetes. For many years, I had been reading the literature on postpartum depression and on the health effects of violence. I had written or edited several books on both topics and always thought of them as separate—until that summer. While working on both topics at the same time, I made an amazing discovery: *I was looking at the same*

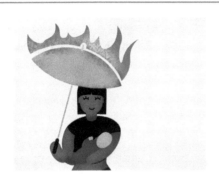

Breastfeeding protects mothers' mental health by lowering inflammation, the physiologic process that underlies depression, anxiety, and posttraumatic stress disorder.

underlying process. It blew my mind (and still does) as I realized that the underlying physiology was the same. More important, it was the first time that I realized that breastfeeding *acted as a powerful physiological agent that protected mothers' mental health.*

The implications of that are huge. It means that when mental health providers discouraged breastfeeding, they were undermining rather than protecting mothers' mental health. Before I describe how breastfeeding benefits mothers, I need to briefly discuss the stress response and the underlying physiology of mental health. Once you know this, the role of breastfeeding will make sense.

UNDERSTANDING THE STRESS RESPONSE

The stress response is key to understanding why breastfeeding protects your mental health. Some of this information will be familiar, but other parts will probably be new. We can consider that the

35

stress response has three main components: catecholamine, the hypothalamic–pituitary–adrenal (HPA) axis, and inflammation (Kendall-Tackett, 2007). All three of these responses help you survive danger, but they can also cause problems when they are on all the time.

Catecholamine (the fight-or-flight response): The catecholamine response is what most people think of as the stress response. As the term *fight-or-flight* implies, it will help you fight your way through a danger (such as when people get super-human strength) or run away. This is the response that happens instantly when your brain perceives danger or threat.

The HPA axis: Researchers documented this system in the late 1990s–early 2000s. As the name implies, there are three structures involved in this response. The three stress hormones from the HPA axis are CRF, ACTH, and cortisol.

The inflammatory-response system: The last component is the inflammatory response system. In response to threat, our bodies increase inflammation. You might wonder why inflammation increases in response to threat or danger. It helps to think about function. Inflammatory molecules fight infection and heal wounds. When you hurt yourself, the area gets hot and red. That's inflammation.

The inflammation response is key in terms of understanding why breastfeeding protects your mental health. Inflammation is the physiological mechanism that underlies depression and other mental health conditions, such as anxiety and posttraumatic stress disorder (PTSD; Bergink et al., 2014; Kendall-Tackett, 2007). When inflammation molecules are high in a person's plasma, they are more likely to be depressed. When they are low, the person is less likely to be depressed (Glaser & Kiecolt-Glaser, 2005; Kiecolt-Glaser et al., 2007). Breastfeeding turns off the inflammation through the work of oxytocin (Groer & Kendall-Tackett, 2011; Uvnäs Moberg, 2015; Uvnäs Moberg et al., 2020).

THE OXYTOCIN RESPONSE

Oxytocin has been called the "love hormone" or the "hormone of attachment." When oxytocin is high, you like other people and want to be around them. You trust them. Oxytocin makes life enjoyable (Uvnäs Moberg, 2013). Oxytocin is released during orgasm, it makes the uterus contract during labor, and it helps you manage labor pain. Oxytocin controls the milk-ejection reflex, when milk lets down, and it helps you cope with the stresses of new motherhood (Uvnäs Moberg, 2015). Oxytocin is the antistress hormone that keeps people healthy throughout their lives.

My friend and colleague Dr. Kerstin Uvnäs Moberg and I have been working together to understand these two systems. Kerstin is a leading expert on oxytocin, and my area is stress and trauma. We realized that our respective areas of research are flip sides of the same coin.

Oxytocin and stress suppress each other. When oxytocin is activated, it suppresses the stress response (including inflammation). Conversely, when the stress system is activated, it suppresses oxytocin. This is why high stress during labor can halt its progress. Stress turns off oxytocin, and oxytocin is necessary for uterine contractions. When a mother is frightened or in extreme pain, stress is activated, and oxytocin is suppressed, and this causes labor to stall (Uvnäs Moberg, 2015) and delays when your milk "comes in," or becomes more abundant (Grajeda & Pérez-Escamilla, 2002).

Dr. Uvnäs Moberg and I came up with a visual to describe the relationship between oxytocin and stress. It's a toggle relationship: When one is up, the other is down. Think of it like a light switch: When the light is on, darkness is suppressed. When the light is off, light is suppressed. Let's now apply this research to both short- and long-term benefits for the mother (Kendall-Tackett, 2007; Uvnäs Moberg, 2015; Uvnäs Moberg et al., 2020).

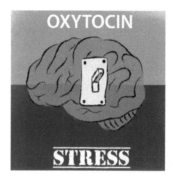

Oxytocin and stress are in a toggle relationship. When one is activated, it suppresses the other. When oxytocin is up, it turns off the stress and inflammatory response and lowers the risk for depression.

SHORT-TERM BENEFITS OF BREASTFEEDING FOR MOTHERS

Breastfeeding lowers mothers' stress almost immediately, as a German study nicely demonstrated. Heinrichs and colleagues (2001) found that nursing immediately lowered mothers' cortisol and ACTH. After mothers nursed and researchers tried to stress them in the lab, the mothers had less of a stress response than they did before they nursed. Breastfeeding appeared to create a lovely little cloud around those mothers for half an hour or so after each time they nursed. Doesn't that make perfect sense? Breastfeeding helps you cope with the stresses of new motherhood. Oxytocin also helps you deal with monotony, which is handy when you're feeding your baby eight to 12 times a day (Uvnäs Moberg, 2015). Heinrichs et al. concluded that breastfeeding provided a short-term lessening of the stress response.

Oxytocin was also at work in a study of 63 first-time mothers at 2 days postpartum (Handlin et al., 2009). Suckling lowered mothers' ACTH levels, and skin-to-skin contact lowered mothers' cortisol.

ACTH and cortisol are often studied because they can be measured in saliva, which is less invasive for the mothers than a blood test to measure inflammation. These hormones are a good way to measure an activated versus nonactivated stress system.

A review from Portugal identified several mechanisms by which breastfeeding can promote mothers' mental health (Figueiredo et al., 2013). When mothers are stressed, breastfeeding lowers the mother's cortisol level. It also regulates mother–infant sleep and helped them feel like more competent mothers.

HEALTH BENEFITS RELATED TO INFLAMMATION

I'm always amazed when people tell me that mothers get no benefit from breastfeeding. I wonder what articles they are reading, because there are many that say the opposite. Let's start with two big benefits: lowered risk of heart disease—the number one killer of women—and its sidekick, diabetes. That should be enough right there, but the same mechanism that lowers risk for these diseases also lowers the risk for depression.

Stuebe et al. (2005) were the first to see this connection. Using data from more than 158,000 nurses, they found that longer duration of breastfeeding reduced the risk of Type 2 diabetes. Each additional year of breastfeeding decreased the risk by 15% even after controlling for known risk factors such as body mass index (BMI), diet, exercise, or smoking. Exclusive breastfeeding reduced risk the most, and longer duration of breastfeeding per pregnancy resulted in greater benefit. For example, there was a stronger effect for nursing one baby for 12 months versus two babies for 6 months each, although all the mothers still benefitted.

Results from the SWAN heart study (Study of Women's Health Across the Nation) included a sample of 2,516 women in midlife (Ram et al., 2008). They found that the longer women breastfed, the lower their risk for metabolic syndrome, a precursor for both heart disease and diabetes. A 2009 study of 139,681 postmenopausal women (mean age = 63) found that women who breastfed had lower lifetime risk of hypertension, diabetes, cardiovascular disease, and high triglycerides (Schwarz et al., 2009). Inflammation is the underlying cause of all of these conditions. The longer women breastfed, the greater the protection, even though many years had passed.

Two Chinese studies had similar findings. The first was a study of 1,260 Chinese women with a history of gestational diabetes (Shen et al., 2019). The researchers found that the more times mothers breastfed each day, and the number of months that they did it, the lower the risk of postpartum diabetes and prediabetes. Similarly, a study of 9,128 Chinese mothers (aged 40–81 years) found that longer breastfeeding was associated with lower risk for hypertension and diabetes even after they controlled for traditional risk factors such waist-to-hip ratio, employment, education, family history, and postpartum BMI (Zhang et al., 2015).

There was a similar finding regarding depression in postmenopausal women. A Korean study (Park & Choi, 2019) included 1,372 postmenopausal mothers who were all older than 50 years. Women who breastfed for at least 47 months (across multiple children) had a 67% decreased risk of postmenopausal depression compared with those who breastfed 0 to 23 months. In addition, there was a 29% decreased risk for each additional infant and a 9% decreased risk for each additional year. Again, these effects occurred many years after breastfeeding and represented lifetime protection.

WHAT HAPPENS WHEN THERE ARE BREASTFEEDING PROBLEMS?

I bet you can answer this one yourself. What happens when you have pain, for example? Is the oxytocin or stress system activated? If you're wounded, your body activates inflammation, and high inflammation means more depression. What if you're constantly worried about your milk supply? Is the stress or the oxytocin system activated? Because researchers often include mothers who are having breastfeeding *problems* in their samples is one reason why there is confusion in the literature.

HOW CAN WE KNOW IT'S BREASTFEEDING THAT PROTECTS MOTHERS' MENTAL HEALTH?

A couple of years ago, I was speaking at a conference and another speaker asked this question. She thought we couldn't tell whether breastfeeding made a difference. She showed a picture of the New York Marathon and asked if running marathons made people healthy or was it that healthier people ran marathons? Let's apply that question to breastfeeding. Are women who breastfeed less likely to be depressed, or are depressed women less likely to breastfeed? Both are actually true. How can we know whether breastfeeding really makes a difference?

This is where the type of study is critical. If you were to use a typical survey (a cross-sectional design), where you go in and only ask the question one time, you could not answer this question because depressed women are less likely to breastfeed (I discuss that in more detail toward the end of this chapter). This means that depressed women will naturally gravitate to the bottle-feeding group. In other words, they self-selected to be in either the breastfeeding or the bottle-feeding groups. Cross-sectional designs can be useful for a lot of research questions, but for this question, they are not helpful at all. Did the mothers' mental state influence her feeding decision? Or did her feeding method influence her mental state? We don't know.

In contrast, a *prospective design* assesses mothers before the study begins and follows them for a length of time. At the beginning

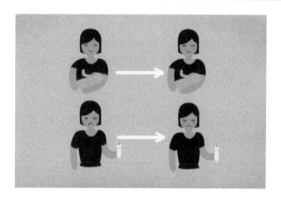

A cross-sectional study of feeding method and mothers' mental health, in which mothers are not assessed for depression at the beginning of the study, cannot tell us whether feeding method makes a difference for maternal mental health because the bottle-feeding mothers are more likely to be depressed at the beginning of the study.

of the study (Time 1), none of the mothers are depressed. By Time 2, we can see whether feeding method makes a difference. If the breast-feeding mothers are less depressed than the bottle-feeding mothers at Time 2, we can reasonably conclude that feeding method did influence mothers' mental health.

Prospective research is generally more expensive and difficult to do, which is why we don't see as much of it. Fortunately, three prospective studies have examined the question of feeding method and mothers' mental health. These studies were all observational (i.e., they didn't include any kind of intervention).

The first prospective study included 2,072 mothers in Sabah, Malaysia (Yusuff et al., 2016). These mothers were studied at 36 to 38 weeks' gestation and at 3 months postpartum. The researchers found significantly less depression (based on scores on the Edinburgh

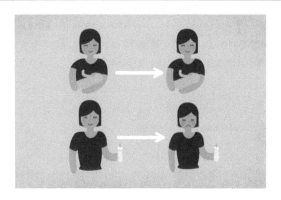

In a prospective study design, mothers' depression is assessed at Time 1, and both groups of mothers are not depressed. By Time 2, it is reasonable to conclude that method makes a difference.

Postnatal Depression Scale) at 3 months postpartum among the mothers who were exclusively breastfeeding.

A prospective study from California included 205 mothers and assessed them five times while they were pregnant and at 3, 6, 12, and 24 months postpartum (Hahn-Holbrook et al., 2013). They found that women who were breastfeeding at 3 months postpartum had significantly lower depression scores at 24 months. They also found that exclusivity made a difference. Women who breastfed nine times a day (exclusive) were significantly less depressed than those who breastfed four times a day (mixed-feeding).

The most recent prospective study was from Portugal and was a prospective study of 334 pregnant women, 70 of whom were depressed and 264 of whom were not depressed (Figueiredo et al., 2021). The researchers assessed women in the third trimester of pregnancy and at 3 to 6 months postpartum and found that for women who were depressed during their pregnancy, exclusive breastfeeding lessened their symptoms and led to lower rates of depression at 3 to 6 months postpartum. They did not find a difference for the mothers who were not depressed during pregnancy.

DEPRESSION, ANXIETY, AND PTSD ARE THREATS TO BREASTFEEDING

There is one more thing to talk about in this chapter, and it's why I've spent the past 25 years talking to lactation professionals about mothers' mental health. If mothers have depression, anxiety, or PTSD, they are less likely to breastfeed. For example, Hahn-Holbrook et al. (2013) found that mothers depressed during pregnancy were less likely to breastfeed and weaned 2.3 months earlier.

A study of mothers who had postpartum anxiety at 3 months postpartum found that they were 11% less likely to exclusively breastfeed at 6 months (Adedinsewo et al., 2014), and I understand why that occurs. Mothers worry about whether their babies are getting enough to eat and offer them a bottle, which they drink right up. Then mothers assume it's because the baby wasn't getting enough to eat from them, rather than that babies take bottles because they're there. Once mothers start down that road, supplementing becomes a regular part of the regimen, which then actually reduces their supply. I've certainly seen this. Anxiety encouraged supplementation, and pretty soon the mothers were no longer exclusively breastfeeding.

Another study looked at women's reasons for stopping breastfeeding when they had mild to severe depression (Bascom & Napolitano, 2016). The reasons for stopping included too many household duties, painful breastfeeding, and exhaustion. All of these reasons indicate that mothers had little support. What would have happened if these mothers had support so that breastfeeding didn't hurt and they weren't so tired? Another study of 2,400 births in the

United States found that women with medically complex pregnancies were 30% less likely to exclusively breastfeed (Kozhimannil et al., 2014). However, supportive hospital practices increased exclusive breastfeeding by 2 to 4 times. Even when mothers face challenges, breastfeeding support (which increases oxytocin) makes a difference.

CONCLUSION

When breastfeeding is going well, it protects maternal mental health by increasing oxytocin and turning off inflammation. High inflammation increases the risk of many mental health problems, including depression, anxiety, and PTSD (Kendall-Tackett, 2017; Maes et al., 2002; Schiepers et al., 2005). Exclusive breastfeeding provides the strongest protection for mental health. Breastfeeding problems, in contrast, can cause depression, anxiety, and trauma symptoms (Brown, 2019; Kendall-Tackett, 2007).

This does not mean that breastfeeding mothers will never get depressed. They certainly can. In fact, I've spent much of my career working with these mothers. But we know that breastfeeding lowers the risk of depression and helps the mother cope while she is in the midst of it. For many mothers, breastfeeding becomes a lifeline, as actor and postpartum depression advocate Brooke Shields (2005) described:

> The consensus seemed to be that I give up the baby on the breast and move past that added pressure. But what nobody understood was that breastfeeding was my only real connection to the baby. If I were to eliminate that, I might have no hope of coming through this nightmare. I was hanging on to the breastfeeding as my lifeline. It was the only thing that made me unique in terms of caring for her, and it created an undeniable connection, even if only a physical one. Without it, she might be lost to me forever. (pp. 80–81)

II

POSITIONING, LATCH, AND NIPPLE PAIN

INTRODUCTION: POSITIONING, LATCH, AND NIPPLE PAIN

Your baby's position at the breast influences how comfortable breast-feeding is for you and how well your baby drinks at the breast. If positioning is off, it will hurt you, and you'll be miserable. If your baby is not drinking milk well, their growth may falter, and it could also interfere with your milk production. Positioning is obviously important, but many mothers worry that they are not doing it "right." Sometimes providers contribute to this. This worries me because I've seen mothers who are so embarrassed about doing it "wrong," that they don't seek help. These mothers suffer for weeks and even months.

I'd like to suspend the idea of right and wrong and talk instead about whether it's working. You'll know it's working if

1. It's not hurting you, and
2. Your baby is drinking well and gaining weight.

The right position is the one that works. Everything else is just noise.

CHAPTER 5

BABY ON YOUR BREAST: POSITIONING, ATTACHMENT, AND BIOLOGICAL NURTURING

Our thinking about positioning has continued to develop over the past 70 years. At the heart of it is whether breastfeeding is instinctual or learned (see Chapter 3). The answer to that question governed how breastfeeding help was provided. This conversation picked up steam when breastfeeding stood on the brink of extinction in the developed world and was at its lowest levels in modern history in the late 1950s and early 1960s. At this point, a couple of generations of mothers had never seen a woman breastfeed. Researchers of the day concluded that women had no instincts with regard to infant feeding and needed to be taught. So began the big push to teach positioning and attachment (P & A).

This instruction did help a lot of mothers, but it was often rigid. Mothers had to sit bolt upright and even lean over their babies to get the "right" latch. Sometimes mothers had their arms out in the air like a chicken wing. We still see this today (it's on a billboard in my neighborhood).

The breastfeeding positions were miserable for a lot of mothers, as it's hard to sit like that for long. Last week, a mother told me that she felt she couldn't move without undoing everything. Unfortunately, very few people can maintain that position for long. If they moved, some mothers said that their health care providers scolded them and told them they were doing it "wrong."

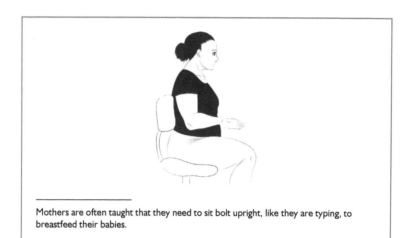

Mothers are often taught that they need to sit bolt upright, like they are typing, to breastfeed their babies.

BIOLOGICAL NURTURING/LAID-BACK BREASTFEEDING

A major shift in this field came from the United Kingdom. Dr. Suzanne Colson, a midwife, observed that standard P & A advice often resulted in sore nipples and ultimately breastfeeding cessation. Through observation and research studies, she developed a paradigm she called Biological Nurturing (BN), also known as "laid-back breastfeeding" (Colson, 2019). In places where it's been implemented, it has revolutionized breastfeeding support. For example, in a recent randomized trial from Italy, 90 postpartum women received breastfeeding support based on BN and 98 received standard care (Milinco et al., 2020). BN substantially reduced the number of breastfeeding problems overall, including cracked and sore nipples, engorgement, and mastitis. At 7 days postpartum, seven mothers had engorgement in the usual care group versus one in the BN group. By 30 days postpartum, there was no significant difference between the groups as mothers in the usual care group improved. By 120 days postpartum, the BN group had a significantly lower number of breastfeeding problems. Unfortunately, even as some of this research is coming out, some professionals resist using BN and so continue to teach standard P & A.

I've used BN with many mothers who had miserably sore nipples, and it usually sorted the problem quickly. The mothers also seem more confident in their abilities to feed and nurture their babies. I know Suzanne quite well. I've worked on both editions of her book, and we've presented together in both Paris and London. Suzanne always says that you can't teach BN, so I'm going to "tell" you about it without (hopefully) too many left-brained instructions (Colson, 2019). I've included a lot of pictures for your right brain.

Sit Comfortably

Pretend that you are watching TV. There is no correct angle here. Your comfort is the most important consideration.

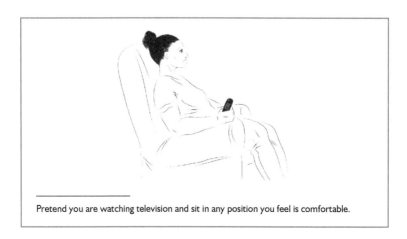

Pretend you are watching television and sit in any position you feel is comfortable.

Have Your Baby at the Right Address

Place your baby face down on your body with your baby's cheek on your breast. Skin-to-skin contact releases oxytocin in you and your baby, and your baby is comforted by smelling your skin and hearing your heartbeat.

Place your baby vertically on your body rather than across your lap. This opens up the space on your body, allows gravity to support your baby's body, and frees up your arms. You don't have to support your baby's weight with your arms because gravity is doing it. With BN, gravity becomes an ally (Colson, 2019).

Watch for Head Bobbing

If your baby is at the right address, you'll know they are hungry when their head starts bobbing up and down. That helps them get to your nipple, and gravity gives them head control. Their hands help find their way to the breast and prepare your breasts for feeding.

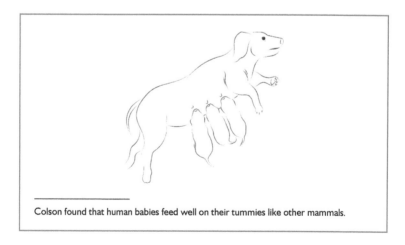

Colson found that human babies feed well on their tummies like other mammals.

When they touch your nipple, it becomes erect and easier to latch on to. When they touch and kneed the breast, it triggers a let-down. Later, when the flow slows, they knead the breast to continue the flow of milk. We've also learned that babies feed well on their tummies, just like other mammals. If you've had a cesarean or don't want baby's feet near your belly, you can drape your baby off to the side. With BN, your baby can be at any angle.

Feel Free to Help

Your baby's reflexes trigger a strong urge in you to help them. Go for it. Mothers' instincts are dormant until they are in the right context. Suzanne documented maternal reflexes. One example is when babies slow their feeding, mothers reach down and stroke the soles of their feet, which encourages suckling (Colson, 2019). Mothers "groom" their babies by stroking the top of their heads, their hands, or their backs. When you see video after video of mothers engaging in the same pattern of behavior, it's pretty convincing.

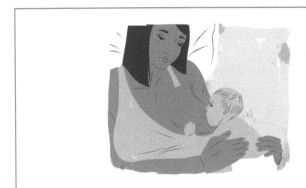

The mother uses her hands around her baby's torso to lift and guide the baby onto her breast.

BN Out and About

You can practice BN when you're out in the world. The key is that the baby is vertical on the mother's body. Discreet BN is even on the front cover of Suzanne's book (Colson, 2019). Once you get the hang of BN, you can adjust to whatever position you like. Soon, you will be confident enough to do it anywhere.

CLASSIC BREASTFEEDING POSITIONS

You may decide that you are more comfortable with the "traditional" breastfeeding positions. Some say these positions are products of the 1950s and 1960s, but you can see them in art, so they are obviously older than that. Millions of women, including me, have successfully breastfed their babies using these positions.

With these positions, you'll notice that there are a lot more instructions. For all of these positions, there are a few basic guidelines:

- *Make sure that there are no gaps between your baby's body and yours.* When gravity pulls the baby's body away from yours, you'll end up with a shallow latch, which will hurt. When using the standard breastfeeding positions, remember "tummy to mummy," with your baby's body in a straight line and their head not turned.
- *Support their feet.* Wrap your baby's body around your own and make sure their feet are supported and are not dangling. If the baby is in an unstable hold, they won't eat. In terms of their reflexes, "not falling" trumps "eating." Sometimes babies compensate for an unstable hold by holding on with their mouths. Ouch!
- *Work with the baby's reflexes.* Babies will still head bob and use their hands, but gravity works against you in this position and pulls your baby away from the breast. Try to work with

those reflexes if you can. Lean back a bit, so your baby has better head control. Remember, head bobbing does not mean that they don't want to nurse. They definitely do.

- *Watch for the early feeding cues.* These include lip-smacking, pulling their fist to their mouth, rooting (nuzzling your breast), or saying "eh, eh, eh." The key is to catch your baby in the early stages of hunger if you can. If they are crying, put them between your breasts to calm them first. You can't cram a breast into a crying baby's mouth. Trying will make you both upset. Calm them down and bring them to your breast again; you're both still figuring it out.

- *Make a nursing station.* Find a comfortable chair with a table nearby. Have your phone, TV remote, a water bottle and snacks, and something to read. This gives you time to relax and enjoy your nursing sessions without needing to get up and grab something you forgot.

Cradle and Cross-Cradle Hold

The cradle hold is one of the most common positions. Some people call this the Madonna position because it appears so often in art.

In this position, you sit on a chair or couch and have the baby across your lap. The baby's head is in the crook of your elbow. The arm you are using is on the same side as your breast. You move your arm to line up with your breast, guiding your baby's head with the crook of your elbow. A lot of people don't use this one because it can be awkward and imprecise.

A somewhat recent variant is the cross-cradle, the position you are more likely to learn in the hospital. With the cross-cradle hold, you use the opposite arm to the breast you are using. Your arm runs the length of the baby's back, and your hand is placed at the back of your baby's head, gently cupping their neck with your fingers at the base of the skull. Avoid touching the back of your baby's head, as

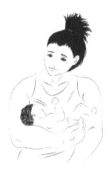

With the cradle position, you guide your baby's head with the crook of your elbow. To keep your arms from getting tired, support them with a pillow.

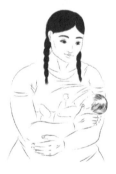

Many mothers prefer the cross-cradle hold because they have better control of the baby's head. Note that the baby's body is in a straight line, and the mother is supporting the baby's head at the base of their skull (not on the back of their head).

this triggers a reflex that makes them move their head backward. Lots of mothers prefer this position to the cradle hold, especially in the early days, because it's easier to control where the baby's head (and mouth) go.

As you are holding your baby across your lap, you may want to put some pillows under the baby to support your arm. It doesn't have to be a special breastfeeding pillow. Those pillows are expensive and frequently the wrong height for many mothers, but if they work for you, that's fine too.

The Football/Rugby Hold

A lot of mothers swear by this position, and it's also great for twins or when you are trying to keep your baby's feet away from a cesarean incision. However, this position doesn't work for every mother, and it depends on the length of your torso and the size of your breasts. With this position, your baby is along your side, supported by your arm, like a football. Your hand is on the base of your baby's skull, so you can use your hand to position your baby.

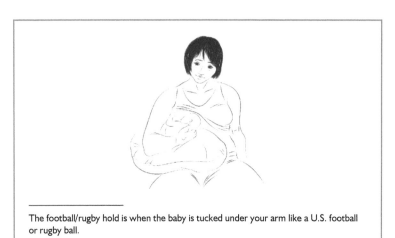

The football/rugby hold is when the baby is tucked under your arm like a U.S. football or rugby ball.

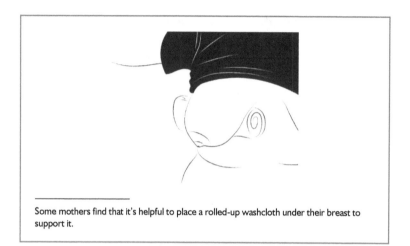

Some mothers find that it's helpful to place a rolled-up washcloth under their breast to support it.

As with the cross-cradle position, use pillows to support your arm so that you do not tire. You can use your free hand to support your breast and guide it.

Be sure to support your baby's feet. Many mothers find that tucking them in with their elbows is helpful. You want to avoid having their feet resting on the chair or sofa back. You'll figure this out pretty quickly as your baby can use that position to push themselves off. Wheeee! So, tuck those little feet in next to your body so you can avoid that.

This position can help if you have large breasts. Some mothers find it helpful to have some extra support by rolling up a washcloth and placing it under your breast.

Side-Lying Position

This position is a great one for you to know and may be the only way for you to get some rest while feeding at night. As with the rest

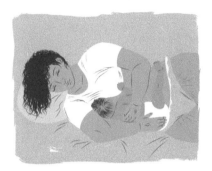

With the side-lying position, your baby is tucked into the nest of your arms, with their whole body facing you.

of the P & A positions, it may take a bit of time for you to master it, but it will be worth the effort. Some mothers find that a rolled-up towel behind the baby's back can keep them in position. Don't use a pillow for safety reasons, as you don't want a pillow near the baby when you're in bed.

In this position, you'll be on your side with your baby on their side facing you when nursing and on their back once they are finished. When it's time to nurse, you scoot your baby near you and roll them onto the breast. You are still going for a deep latch, and you may need to use your hand to shape your breast, especially in the beginning (see the breast sandwich in the next section).

SOME HANDY TRICKS

There are a couple of tricks that can get your baby comfortably on your breast for an effective latch.

The Breast Sandwich

A video demonstrating how to use the breast sandwich.

This helpful tip originally came from New York lactation consultant Diane Wiessinger (1998). Picture yourself eating a sandwich that is too big for your mouth. What do you do? You shape the sandwich, so it fits. In the same way, you can shape your breast so that your baby can latch. This is particularly helpful if you have a full or round breast. By making a breast sandwich, you make a firmer surface, which can also help your baby if they are struggling because your breast is soft and is larger than your baby's mouth.

In the early days, you may need to hold this position for the whole time they feed. However, you may only need to do this while they latch. If you let go and they start to slip, you may need to relatch them.

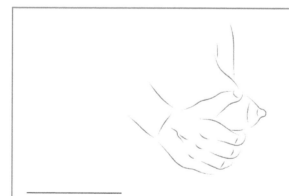

The breast sandwich allows you to shape your breast so that it's easier for your baby to latch.

I've shown quite a few mothers how to do this. In some cases, it can make the difference between a latching and nonlatching baby. It can also be helpful when mothers are engorged, have sore nipples, or have flat or inverted nipples (it gives a more solid surface for the babies to latch).

The Asymmetrical Latch and the Flipple

Early on, we assumed that the nipple needed to be centered in the baby's mouth like a bullseye with an equal amount of lip on either side. In the past 20 years, we learned that an effective latch is asymmetrical, meaning that the lower jaw needs to be deeper on the breast than the top jaw. The lower jaw is the one that does all the work in bringing the milk forward to your baby, while the top jaw doesn't move. If the bottom jaw is too close to your nipple, every time it moves, it smashes your nipple against your baby's hard pallet. You'll get a crease across your nipple, or it will look like lipstick when it comes out of your baby's mouth. It will also hurt like mad.

Here's a trick to get an asymmetrical latch. Place your baby's chin on your breast first. That will trigger them to open their mouth wide. Line your baby's nose up with your nipple. Once they open wide, you can roll your baby on to the rest of the breast or simply "flip" your nipple into their mouth (the "flipple"), a term Australian lactation consultant Rebecca Glover (n.d.) coined.

Don't worry if you don't have the whole areola in, as it may be larger than your baby's mouth. As long as they have a deep latch, it doesn't matter. Your baby will close their mouth and begin to suckle. You should hear swallowing. It will sound like "caw, caw, caw."

If your baby is sleepy or reluctant to open their mouth, you can squeeze a few drops of breast milk out to encourage them to open wide.

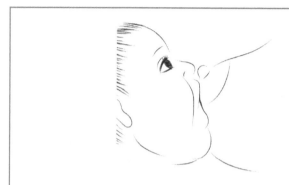

Place your baby's chin on your breast first. This will signal them to open their mouth wide. From there, you can rock your baby onto your breast or simply flip your nipple into their mouth ("the flipple").

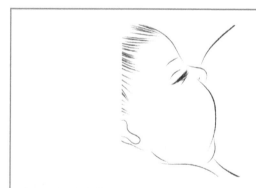

With a deep latch, your baby's cheeks and chin are against your breast. You should hear audible swallowing, and it should not hurt (although you might have a small twinge when you first start). If it's more than a small twinge, break the seal and try again.

A video demonstrating the Flipple for latching your baby on to your breast.

If your baby latches and it hurts, gently release the latch and try again. When releasing the latch, insert your pinky into the corner of their mouth to break the seal. If you don't do that first, it will hurt, and you will damage your nipple in the process.

If your baby gets upset or is screaming, stop what you are doing and use your body to calm your baby down by placing them vertically between your breasts. If your baby is still crying, try putting them a little higher on your body. Many babies like that better. The main thing is to calm them down. You want your baby to feel happy at your breast not hysterical and unhappy. If you calm your baby first, they are less likely to associate your breast with an unhappy place.

You might also be getting frustrated or upset. It's not unusual to have a screaming baby and a crying mother. Be gentle with both of you. You're both learning and will get the hang of it soon. If you're

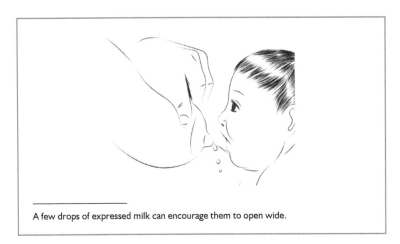

A few drops of expressed milk can encourage them to open wide.

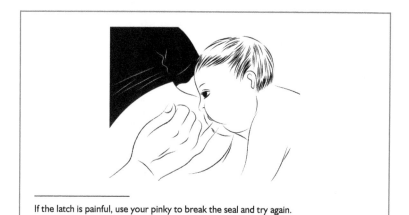

If the latch is painful, use your pinky to break the seal and try again.

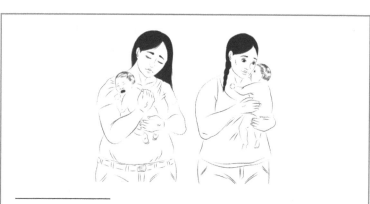

When babies are too low on their parents' bodies, they are often upset. Placing your baby a little higher on your body so that they can peer over your shoulder usually calms them down.

really struggling with getting your baby to latch, express some milk and feed them a bit before you try latching them on, just enough to take the edge off their hunger. (See the next section.)

If you are struggling—or have any questions at all—please reach out to a peer supporter or lactation specialist. If it's painful and they tell you that "the latch looks fine" or it's "normal" to have pain, please see someone else. They're not giving you good advice.

MY BABY DOESN'T LIKE ME

It's heartbreaking when a mother tells me that her baby screams, arches, or pushes away every time she brings them to her breast. She often concludes that her baby doesn't like breastfeeding—or worse, doesn't like her. This belief can crush a new mother.

Reasons Why Babies May Resist Breastfeeding

Before we go further, I want to tell you that your baby loves you best of all. Your baby knows your voice and your smell. Your body comforts them. But in your right-brain state, you may not believe it. So I'm going to talk to your left brain as we try to figure out what is going on. This isn't, strictly speaking, a latch issue, but it definitely affects your baby's feeding at the breast. Your baby resisting the breast does not reflect how your baby feels about you. **Repeat after me: "My baby is NOT rejecting me. This is a breastfeeding problem, and we will solve it."**

Let's go through some common reasons why babies resist the breast.

DID SOMEONE TRY TO FORCE YOUR BABY TO BREASTFEED?

This is one of the most common reasons why babies get upset at the breast. Someone at the hospital tried to "help" by shoving your baby onto the breast. Babies don't like that, and they quickly learn that the breast is not a happy place to be. It's standard classical conditioning (think Pavlov's dog) pairing an activity (breastfeeding) with something negative (being forced to the breast).

SLOW MILK FLOW AT THE BREAST

Some babies become frustrated at the breast when the flow of milk is slow. It could be due to low supply or delayed lactogenesis II (LG II; see Chapter 8), or they got used to the faster flow from a bottle. A hungry baby can get quickly cranky and will let you know. Breast compressions help. You can also use a pump to get milk flowing before your latch your baby.

FAST FLOW AT THE BREAST

Babies may reject the breast when you have a lot of milk, and it comes out quickly. If they are in the cradle, cross-cradle, or football (rugby) hold, they can't get away from it. Laid-back breastfeeding helps because gravity slows the flow of milk and babies can lift their heads to get away from it and latch back on once it slows.

A friend from California called me when their fourth baby was arching and pulling away from the breast, but only on the left side. When the milk started to flow, he was using both hands to push away. Mom and Dad couldn't figure out what was going on. I thought he might be responding to a fast flow. The mom used a pump to get the milk flowing so it slowed a bit before latching him to that side.

BABY WAS INJURED AT BIRTH

Some birth injuries are serious and obvious, such as a broken arm or collarbone. Some are more subtle, such as shoulders or ribs that are sore and miserable, and it hurts when they lie on their left (or right) side. They are not rejecting YOU, but they are letting you know that it hurts to be in that position.

WHAT TO DO

The overwhelming majority of babies go back to the breast. Every once in a while, you have a baby who will not latch, but they are the exception. The goal is to help your baby (and you) be happy at the breast. Some of their advice is similar to what we've already discussed but in a different context.

Make the Breast a Happy Place to Be

Thinking about the principles of classical conditioning, you want your baby to associate your breast with happy things. If they are frustrated, hungry, or in pain, they form the opposite association and don't want to go back. Everyone ends up in tears. It's a bad situation all around.

A lovely friend called me at 7 a.m. one morning and asked, "Is this a good time to talk?" I knew something was up. She had a hard time getting her baby to feed in the middle of the night and wanted to know if it was okay for her to use a bottle of expressed milk for that feed. I said, "absolutely." They continued to work on latch that morning, and he happily nursed for several months. The most important thing in that moment at 3 a.m. was getting the baby fed. We want baby and mom happy.

For reluctant nursers, Dr. Tina Smillie suggests a "bait-and-switch" technique. While holding your baby against your breast, give them a short bottle feed to take the edge off their hunger and then slide them on to the breast. If they get frustrated, stop and try again with another feeding.

PICK UP ON EARLY FEEDING CUES

Figuring out breastfeeding is easier when everyone is calm. If you can catch your baby in the earliest stages of hunger, you have a better chance of getting them to take the breast. As I mentioned previously, early cues include lip-smacking, bringing their fist to their mouths, rooting, and saying "eh, eh, eh." You won't always catch these, but if you can, the early days will be easier.

CALM YOUR BABY BEFORE BRINGING THEM TO BREAST

Say you've missed the early cues or your baby is one of those who goes from 0 to 60 and skips the early cues altogether. In this case, don't try to bring your baby to breast yet. Take a minute and calm your baby down with your body. Hold your baby upright between your breasts and make gentle shushing noises. When you can comfort your baby with your body, it clearly indicates that your baby is not rejecting *you*. Also, your baby will learn to associate your body with comfort, which is what we want.

FEED THEM WHILE THEY SLEEP

This strategy works well and can also be used when older babies go on a nursing strike (suddenly refuse to breastfeed after weeks or months of breastfeeding well). Try latching them when they are in light sleep (you'll see fluttery eyelids).

NURSE STANDING UP

Sometimes a change from sitting to standing can persuade a reluctant nurser to latch.

USE BODY WORK

If you think that your baby might have an injury, or if they seem to cry a lot, an infant chiropractor or craniosacral therapist can help (Berg-Drazin, 2019; Miller, 2019). Both of these modalities are very gentle. When they start feeling better, it will be easier for them to nurse.

CONCLUSION

Breastfeeding comfortably and without pain can be challenging in the beginning, but comfort determines whether you'll continue. Most of the time, breastfeeding problems are solvable, but the challenge is finding a provider who will assess you and suggest things you can try. Unfortunately, some providers still think they are "supporting breastfeeding" by telling you everything is "fine." You will know when things are not working. In the next chapter, I'll describe things that contribute to breast pain and what you can do to address them.

CHAPTER 6

SORE NIPPLES AND ENGORGEMENT

Breast and nipple pain are extraordinarily common. In our survey, 57% of mothers reported nipple pain, and our findings are consistent with previous studies. A study from Minneapolis found that 50% of women had nipple pain at 5 weeks postpartum (McGovern et al., 2006). In Toronto, 52% had nipple pain at 2 months (Ansara et al., 2005), and 60% had pain in a study from Lithuania (Leviniene et al., 2013). Although nipple pain is common, it is not normal. "Common" means lots of people experience it. "Normal" means that it's part of everyday breastfeeding. It's not, nor should it be. In this chapter, I describe both engorgement, which tends to happen fairly early in the postpartum period, and nipple pain, which can occur at any time and persist for days or even weeks.

ENGORGEMENT

> I had severe engorgement of breasts on third and fourth day even though I had started breastfeeding in the first few hours after the birth of my baby. I had to express my milk to loosen my breast so that baby can easily latch on my breast. Otherwise, there were no problems. (Mother in our survey)

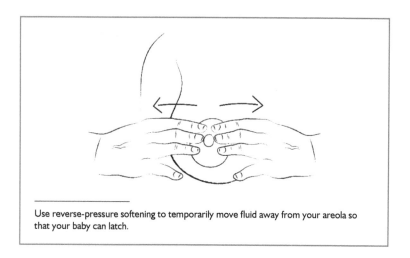

Use reverse-pressure softening to temporarily move fluid away from your areola so that your baby can latch.

Engorgement happens to many women around Day 3 to 4. Your breasts become inflamed and hot to the touch, with a dramatic increase in size. You'll want to address this immediately because it is painful and can halt or slow milk production. Babies also have a hard time latching while you are engorged, which can intensify the problem. Engorgement is caused by an increase in milk and in blood and lymphatic fluid. The goal is to reduce inflammation and swelling as quickly as possible.

Reverse-Pressure Softening

Reverse-pressure softening (RPS) was a technique developed by lactation consultant Jean Cotterman (2004). To use RPS, put your fingers around the outside edges of your areola and press toward your chest wall to move fluid from your

A video demonstration of reverse-pressure softening.

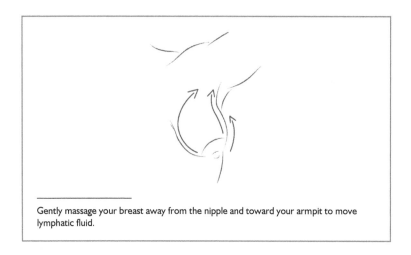

Gently massage your breast away from the nipple and toward your armpit to move lymphatic fluid.

areola, up higher into your breast, so that your body can eventually move it out and get rid of it. The primary goal is to move fluid from around your nipple so your baby can latch.

Lymphatic Drainage

A video demonstration of lymphatic drainage for engorgement.

Lymphatic drainage is a technique that can work well to move fluid out of your breasts. Your lymphatic system is near your skin, so you only need gentle massage; hard strokes don't work and are counterproductive. Use lotion or corn starch on your hands so they glide on your skin. You can do this, or someone can help you. Make gentle upward strokes away from your nipple toward your armpit. Your armpit has a lot of lymph nodes that will move that fluid out of your body. I learned this technique from lactation consultant Maya Bolman, who learned it from her grandmother, a midwife in Ukraine. After watching Maya's videos, I was amazed by how quickly it worked and how much relief it provided. You can do this until the engorgement resolves.

Cold Packs

Applying a cold pack to your breasts can also reduce inflammation. You can use a gel cold pack (available where you buy ACE or tensor bandages) or a pack of peas. Don't leave cold packs on for longer than 20 minutes at a time because they can irritate your skin.

Green Cabbage Leaves

This is a folk remedy that some mothers like. You chill a green cabbage, take off a leaf, crunch it in your hand, and wrap it around your breast under your bra. Remove and discard once it gets warm. The cool leaf is soothing and crunching the leaf releases a substance that is purported to help with the inflammation, although some mothers found it irritating.

Anti-Inflammatories

It's okay to take an anti-inflammatory medication such as ibuprofen while you are engorged. It will reduce inflammation while also relieving pain.

Breastfeed Frequently but Pump Sparingly

Frequent feeding helps reduce the pressure in your breasts. Some mothers also pump while engorged. You can pump to make yourself more comfortable, but try not to drain your breasts because this extra removal can signal your body to make more milk, which could inadvertently make the problem worse.

NIPPLE PAIN

As I described in the introduction to this chapter, nipple pain is common around the world. Yet mothers are often given poor advice about it. Practitioners, and some groups on Facebook and other social media, may tell you that it's just a part of breastfeeding. Many of them experienced it, so it must be "normal." Unfortunately, these groups conflate "common" with "normal." It is common (i.e., it happens to a lot of people), but it is definitely not normal. Our body uses pain to tell us to stop. We are not "supporting" a mother in pain by telling her that she should "keep doing what you are doing" or that the "latch looks fine" if she is in pain. That's telling her to walk with the rock in her shoe and is, in my opinion, poor practice. Here's what one mother in our survey said:

> The latch was very painful, but [the] lactation consultant told me it looked perfect. I was given a nipple shield, but it didn't help much, so I tried it off and on in the first few weeks before discarding it. Pain became bearable in about 2 weeks, and we eventually got it figured out on our own.

Not surprisingly, pain can influence mothers' mental health. In one study, breast pain at Day 1, Week 1, or Week 2 was related to increased risk of depression at 2 months (Watkins et al., 2011). However, if the mothers had breastfeeding help, just having help protected mothers' mental health if they had moderate or severe pain. If I were to hypothesize why this might be so, I'd say it's likely an effect of oxytocin. Social support increases oxytocin and lowers inflammation, which protects their mental health (Uchino et al., 2018). Even when they experienced pain, they knew that help was near.

Sometimes when a mother has pain, the problem is something we can quickly fix. Other times we may need to try several things, but for the mothers I've worked with, it has always gotten better, even when the problem has gone on for a while. Let me give you an example. I met Lee in the north of England. She had been suffering with painful breastfeeding for 7 *weeks* and had made the rounds to her midwife and some mother-to-mother support organizations. The midwives told her she shouldn't have pain because the latch looked "fine" (pain is a good indicator that it is not fine!). The mother-to-mother group wasn't much better. Amazingly, this mother persisted. I met her out in the waiting room while the breastfeeding peer supporters were having a meeting. I chatted with her while her baby slept and realized that she needed help pronto. When her baby woke up, I watched her nurse, I could see immediately that the baby was too far away from her body and was not supported. Breastfeeding was painful because he was hanging on with his mouth. Ouch!

With her permission, I got behind her and guided her hands to get the baby closer. I showed her how to hold her breast like a sandwich so her baby could latch. He latched immediately, and she said, "Oh my God, that doesn't hurt." The baby immediately started loudly gulping, and the mother said, "Wow! He's never done that before." She was thrilled. I saw her the next day at the conference, and breastfeeding was still going well.

In retrospect, I wonder how all the people who saw her nurse could think that the latch was "fine." The positioning was off, and the mother told them she was in pain (over and over). Those providers needed to do a proper evaluation and find out what was going on. Instead, they blew her off. I was extremely proud of this mom for persisting, but I worried that this experience had affected her mental health.

As I've thought about this issue, I've realized that we in the lactation field need to work on our messaging around nipple pain. Sometimes people will say, "Breastfeeding should be completely pain-free," but if mothers read that, and they're experiencing pain, they think "I'm doing it wrong." Here's my take. I believe that breast-feeding should be pain-free. However, I know that it can hurt in the early days for many reasons, not just how you're doing it. You might be tender. There could be something structural in the baby's mouth or an infection. Our goal is to figure out what is going on so that it no longer hurts.

Troubleshooting Nipple Pain

As a general rule, seek professional support if you are in pain. If none is available, or if you are told that everything is "fine," I've listed here the most common reasons why you might have nipple pain.

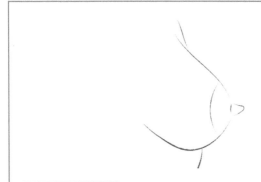

If your nipple is shaped like lipstick, with the bottom of your nipple at a diagonal, it means that your baby's bottom jaw is too close to your nipple. Every time your baby sucks, they smash your nipple against their hard pallet. Moving your baby's jaw deeper on the breast pulls your nipple further back into their mouths so that it doesn't get injured.

LATCH/POSITIONING/ATTACHMENT

Video demonstrating the effects of a shallow latch on your nipple.

A shallow latch is the most common culprit. If your nipple comes out of your baby's mouth with a crease across your nipple or your nipple is shaped like a lipstick, your baby's jaw is too near the nipple.

Some mothers find that nipple pain spontaneously improves at about 6 weeks. When that happens, it's usually because the baby has more head control and can adjust themselves on the breast. Six weeks is *way* too long for you to wait.

WHY BABIES MAY HAVE A SHALLOW LATCH

1. *Positioning.* There are gaps between you and your baby's body; your baby's body may not be facing you, or their head may be turned.
2. *"OBD."* This is something my friend Diana West calls "oral-boobular disproportion." In other words, not a good match between the size of your breast and your baby's mouth. This doesn't mean that your breast, or nipple, is "too big," but it could be that your baby has a tiny mouth, and your nipple doesn't quite fit—yet! Time will change that. This may especially be an issue if your baby was a little early. The breast sandwich helps a lot. Hand-expressing some colostrum onto a spoon can also help in the early days.
3. *Your baby's anatomy.* Your baby may have a slight jaw recession, meaning that it sits back a bit from their top lip. That's perfectly normal, and it gives them their "baby face," but it can make it harder for them to latch. As they mature, their

jaw moves forward. In the meantime, using the laid-back position can help because it brings your baby's jaw forward. The breast sandwich helps here too.

4. *Your anatomy.* You may have flat or inverted nipples, or your breast may be too soft for your baby to hold on to. Most mothers with flat nipples can breastfeed successfully, but a nipple shield may help them get a deeper latch. As your baby matures, you usually can wean yourself off of the shield. Some mothers with flat or inverted nipples find that using a nipple everter (a device that temporarily pulls the nipple out) or a Supple Cup before bringing their babies to their breast helps their babies get a deep latch without a shield, and using the breast sandwich gives them a firmer surface.

5. *Tongue-tie.* Tongue-tie can also cause sore nipples. Please review the section on tongue-tie later in this chapter and have this evaluated. Sometimes all it takes is a simple snip to make all the difference. One possible indicator of tongue-tie is the baby making clicking sounds at the breast. A tongue-tie isn't a problem if it's not hurting you and your baby is getting enough to eat. If it's hurting, have it evaluated. Sometimes laid-back positioning helps because it draws the tongue forward (Colson, 2019).

If Your Latch Is Shallow

- *Review the previous chapter on latch and put your baby vertically on your body rather than across your lap.*
- *If you think your baby is on you too shallowly, insert your pinky in the corner of your baby's mouth to break the seal, then try again.*
- *Make sure your baby is snuggled up completely against you with no gaps between your bodies.* If you are using one of the sitting positions, try bringing your baby's nose level with your nipple (to ensure that the lower jaw is further from the nipple), put the baby's chin on your breast and rock their mouth on to the breast.

- *Try using the breast sandwich to help your baby latch more deeply.*

If your baby is frustrated and screaming, calm them down before you try again. A bit of milk first in a bottle or cup may take the edge off before you try again.

INFECTION

I've met mothers in excruciating pain because of a yeast or bacterial infection. Signs of a yeast infection are red, shiny skin on your nipples and areolas (Khan & Ritchie, 2019). Another possible sign is white patches in your baby's mouth (although you may not always see these). If you're not sure, you could try an over-the-counter antifungal, such as nystatin or Gentian violet. Be sure to gently wipe it off before you bring your baby to your breast. Your baby's provider can also treat them for a fungal infection at the same time that you are being treated.

Bacterial infections are also painful. *Staphylococcus aureus* is the most common type of infection, and it is more likely if there is a breach in your skin (like a cracked nipple). If your breast is hot, has red streaks, or has visible pus in the wound, call your health care provider ASAP, especially if you have a fever or are achy (Khan & Ritchie, 2019). Don't play around with infection, because it's painful and can cause an abscess. Also be sure that you are emptying your breast regularly (via baby or pump) and you've had someone evaluate your baby's latch and mouth to see what is damaging your nipple.

VASOSPASM OR RAYNAUD'S PHENOMENON

Raynaud's phenomenon refers to a temporary vasospasm that cuts off blood flow to an extremity, such as your fingers and toes (Khan & Ritchie, 2019). A vasospasm is a brief narrowing of blood vessels that restricts blood flow. The body part affected will be cold to the touch and may turn white or blue. Raynaud's can also affect your nipples. If your nipples look white after they come out of your baby's mouth, that could be a sign of Raynaud's.

Raynaud's can be caused by repeated nipple damage, so that your breasts react with a spasm. Cold, stress, or an underlying condition, such as an autoimmune disease, can also trigger it. Raynaud's causes acute pain. If you walk into someplace cold, you may feel a stabbing pain in your breasts. Here are some ways to deal with it.

- *Address latch issues because a shallow latch can cause vasospasm in the nipples.*
- *Avoid cold exposure while breastfeeding.* A cold draft can cause a spasm. Keep yourself warm, stay away from drafts, and possibly wrap something warm around your shoulders while you nurse.
- *Raise your core body temperature.* I've lived with Raynaud's most of my adult life; raising my core temperature usually helps, which you can do by drinking something hot. Have a cup of hot tea before you nurse (for safety reasons, don't drink something hot while holding your baby). Keeping yourself warm while breastfeeding also helps.
- *Protect your breasts from cold.* If you are having cold weather or walk into a cold room, put your arm across your breasts to protect them from the blast of cold air.
- *Take medication.* You generally do not need medical care for Raynaud's, but if your symptoms are severe, you can try taking a calcium-channel blocker like nifedipine.

PUMP PROBLEMS

A pump flange that is too tight can injure your nipples. You need a flange that is snug enough to create suction from the pump but not so tight that your nipple is banging against the sides. Your nipple will

83

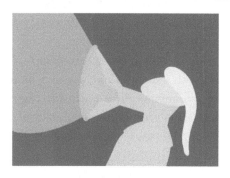

Make sure that your nipple is not too close to the sides of the flange. There needs to be room for your nipple to expand while pumping but not so much space that there is no suction.

swell in the pump, so you want a flange to accommodate the increase in size when you are pumping. The safest bet is to have someone evaluate this, especially if you have large nipples and are experiencing soreness. You may need a bigger flange.

Overvigorous pumping can also damage your nipples. Use enough suction to remove milk but not so much that it's hurting you. If it hurts to pump, try lowering the setting. More is not always better. If you're in pain, your body will shut down oxytocin, making it more difficult for you to get any milk from your breasts (oxytocin is necessary for milk ejection).

Pumping problems can also be caused by a bad pump. Many mothers find that battery-operated pumps cause pain (but some have great luck with them). If you need to pump a lot, your best bet is either a hospital-grade pump or a single-user double-electric pump, such as Pump-in-Style or Purely Yours. If you're hurting and using a cheap pump, consider upgrading. In the United States, you probably qualify for one through the Affordable Care Act, WIC, or your insurer. It's worth checking into.

TONGUE-TIE

> I wish they would've diagnosed a lip/tongue tie in the hospital. It would've saved so much pain and suffering, not to mention weight loss.

> The ENT saw me straight away and released the tongue. We never had the breastfeeding experience I dreamed of . . . I was triple feeding until he was 6 months [feeding at the breast, pumping, and then feeding the pumped milk with a bottle]. I was exhausted and spiraling into depression. I attended your session at ILCA [International Lactation Consultant Association] conference in 2010 in San Antonio as was able to identify some of my feelings and experience based off your conference session. I knew immediately I wanted to be an IBCLC [International Board Certified Lactation Consultant] to help moms.

Tongue-tie can also cause sore nipples and other breastfeeding problems. It's caused by a small piece of connective tissue that connects the tongue to the floor of the mouth, restricting movement so that your baby can't cup their tongue under the breast or move their tongue to remove milk. It causes problems with both shallow latch and milk removal. I'm discussing this separately because there is so much controversy around this topic.

When I collected mothers' stories about tongue-tie for a round-table discussion we were publishing, the stories had a lot in common: (a) weeks or months in pain, (b) babies "on all the time," (c) faltering weight gains, and (d) no one was listening to them. Mothers found the information they needed from other mothers and became evangelical themselves regarding tongue-tie revisions. Some sites even diagnose via Facebook. I understand that these mothers are trying to spare others from pain and suffering, but tongue-tie needs to be evaluated in person by a professional.

Signs of Possible Tongue-Tie

- *A band of tissue that restricts the movement of the tongue.*
  Lift your baby's tongue and you may see a web of tissue. That
  could be a tongue-tie, but it may not be a problem if babies can
  stick out their tongue over their bottom lip. I had someone tell
  me I had a tongue-tie even though I can stick out my tongue,
  eat an ice cream cone, and play the clarinet. In other words,
  it hasn't been a problem. If it's not hurting you, and your
  baby is drinking milk, don't worry about it. If it is causing
  problems, have someone evaluate it.
- *Clicking at the breast.* If your baby is making clicking sounds
  while at the breast, or seems to pull on and off, get it evaluated.
  If it's not hurting, and your baby is getting enough to eat, you
  should be fine.
- *Tongue is heart shaped.* Sometimes, a tongue-tie will cause your
  baby's tongue to appear heart shaped because it's pulling in the
  middle. Lack of heart shape doesn't mean it's not a tongue-tie
  (again, get it evaluated), but this can be a sign.

How to Treat

There are two types of tongue-tie: anterior and posterior.

ANTERIOR TIE

An anterior tie is one that is toward the front of the tongue and is
the easiest to address. It's usually just a simple snip of the frenulum
(the tissue holding the tongue). The procedure is called a frenotomy.
It sounds awful, but it doesn't seem to hurt the babies, although they
do get mad when they are being held down. It usually doesn't bleed
more than a drop or two (if at all), and no sutures are needed.

I became convinced about the efficacy of frenotomy after seeing before-and-after ultrasounds of babies at the breast (Garbin et al., 2013). They showed milk transfer before and after the procedure. Mothers reported that it was immediately better, but if tongue-tie was not diagnosed right away, the baby may need some therapy that can help retrain the tongue.

POSTERIOR TIE

The more controversial procedure is surgery to correct a posterior tie, a tie at the back of the tongue. Practitioners diagnose it by mother's history and by feeling for a bump at the back of the tongue. This procedure is more involved and includes surgery and sutures. I originally didn't know too much about it but got pulled into the controversy because a couple of my friends had been targeted by a particularly aggressive Facebook group. I followed the link and was amazed by what I saw.

I also became concerned about this procedure when several colleagues whose opinions I trust, and who have been at the forefront of tongue-tie work, privately expressed concern that things might have gone too far. A pediatrician-IBCLC told me that she had seen some pretty miserable babies who had had posterior revisions. She wished they had explored more conservative options first. On the other hand, I'd be remiss if I didn't tell you that some mothers and babies have had great outcomes from posterior revisions.

If you are considering a posterior revision for your baby, I'd strongly encourage you to read our *Expert Roundtable on Tongue-tie* as it will give you both sides and allow you to make an informed decision (Kendall-Tackett, Walker, & Genna, 2018). It's on Kindle, too, so you can get it right away. I will briefly summarize the controversy around posterior ties here, but it's worth reading the full report. Revision of a posterior tie is much more involved than a revision for an anterior tie. With the anterior tie, revision is a quick snip with surgical scissors. For a posterior tie, it is an incision on the bottom of the tongue, often done with a laser, and it needs stitches. Sometimes the harm caused by the procedure outweighs the benefit. Dr. Carmela Baeza shared a case study in our roundtable on an infant whose mouth had been badly burned by a laser and was now refusing to eat (Kendall-Tackett, Walker, & Genna, 2018). Other practitioners have shared similar stories of babies who have had multiple revisions that did not improve outcomes.

After surgery, some practitioners recommend stretching exercises for the tongue so that scar tissue does not form. The stretching exercises are also controversial because many parents (and babies) do not like having to do them. Dr. James Murphy says that you need these exercises to prevent scars from forming, but Dr. Tina Smillie says that these exercises fly in the face of everything we know about wound healing. These are both practitioners whom I respect, and both have had good results treating tongue-tie (Kendall-Tackett, Walker, & Genna, 2018).

The final issue is evidence. Although we have research that supports clipping anterior ties, we do not have empirical evidence that supports revisions of posterior ties. We have clinical evidence, with some practitioners reporting good outcomes, but that's not the same. It's not unusual in a clinical field that clinical evidence proceeds research evidence, but it suggests that you may want to learn more about it before you proceed to judge whether the possible benefit is worth the risk.

A Couple of Other Things to Try Before a Posterior Revision

- *Craniosacral therapy (CST)*. CST is a type of energy or mind–body medicine that can be helpful. Some people, especially online, are skeptical about CST and think it's rubbish. (If you read articles online, they are pretty forthright.) If you are skeptical about CST, you might want to avoid it as your beliefs about a treatment's efficacy influence whether it actually works for you. Fortunately, you have other choices that may feel more comfortable. If you want to give CST a try, it may work well for you.

CST may help because it can realign the bones in your baby's skull. Unlike adult skulls, the bones in a baby's head are held together by connective tissue, which allows the head bones to be malleable so that they fit in the birth canal. Birth can subtly knock these out of alignment, which can cause feeding difficulties (Berg-Drazin, 2019). CST is extremely gentle. You will know in a session or two if it's going to help. Although this is not evidence, I've had personal experience with this modality after a car accident. It eliminated a painful problem and did so in a way that didn't really fit into the framework of Western medicine. Several of the practitioners in our roundtable recommended CST as a modality to try (Kendall-Tackett, Walker, & Genna, 2018).

- *Infant chiropractic.* Infant chiropractic is another technique to try. Dr. Joyce Miller (2019) is one of the best sources on chiropractic on infants. She has trained practitioners all over the world. Infant chiropractic is also extremely gentle. It too can help gently move joints in your baby's face and head that may have been out of alignment from birth. When things are lined up the way they are supposed to be, it will be more comfortable for you to nurse, and your baby will feel better too. In Dr. Miller's book *Evidence-Based Chiropractic Care for Infants*, she summarizes the results of numerous randomized trials demonstrating the efficacy of chiropractic for infants. Chiropractic also helps when babies cry a lot. If you want to know more, her book is a great resource.

WHAT TO DO WHILE YOUR NIPPLES HEAL

These measures are not a substitute for addressing the underlying cause of sore nipples. Be sure to do that too, preferably by seeing a lactation specialist.

- *Purified lanolin.* This has become oddly controversial in the lactation world. Some of my colleagues believe that sending mothers home from the hospital with lanolin tells them that nipple pain is normal. You know my position on that (that it's common, not normal). If you have damage, lanolin can ease the pain while promoting moist wound healing and keeping you from scabbing. Be sure to get the purified lanolin, like Lansinoh. Most chains, such as Walmart, carry this. You don't need to wash it off before you nurse.
- *Hydrogel dressings.* Many mothers report that these help with pain immediately, especially if they are chilled. They protect the damaged skin and facilitate moist healing. The risk of infection is low, which is important when there is a cut or opening in the skin (Dodd & Chalmers, 2003).
- *Over-the-counter pain medication.* It's okay to take something like ibuprofen or acetaminophen to make you feel better. Those medications are compatible with breastfeeding.
- *APNO.* APNO stands for all-purpose nipple ointment and was developed by Canadian pediatrician and lactation consultant Dr. Jack Newman. Many mothers swear by it. It contains an antibiotic, steroid, and antifungal and can be obtained at a compounding pharmacy. You can find more information on Dr. Newman's web page in the reference list in the back of this book (Newman, n.d.-a).
- *Pump/hand express until you heal.* If there's a lot of nipple damage, you may need to temporarily stop feeding at the breast and pump to give your nipples a chance to heal and maintain

your supply. Use your milk to feed the baby. It should improve in a day or two but take the time you need. Also, if you are using a pump, make sure that your pump flanges are not too tight as that can cause nipple damage too. Hand expression also works well and won't damage your nipples. Be sure to empty your breasts at least eight times a day.

TREATMENTS FOR SORE NIPPLES THAT DON'T WORK

Some mothers have their efforts scuttled by advice that doesn't fix the problem. Here are two of the most common.

Lanolin Without Addressing the Underlying Problem

Lanolin has gotten a bad rep because practitioners sometimes use it as a "treatment" for sore nipples. It won't work if you don't fix the underlying problem. It's like using a Band-Aid (plaster) after surgery. Lanolin can help nipples heal, but you need to keep them from being reinjured first.

Nipple Shields

These can be useful for some specific situations (like inverted nipples or with a small preterm baby). They do not help with sore nipples, and if the underlying problem is not addressed, your nipple will continue to be injured. One recent study found that when mothers were using nipple shields for pain, babies still got enough milk, but the nipple shields did not lessen the pain (Coentro et al., 2021).

IF YOU'RE STILL HAVING PAIN

The causes of nipple pain listed in the previous section cover most mothers. However, if you are still having pain, there may be something else going on anatomically. For example, your baby may have a high palate. If this is the case, a specialist can identify the problem. You might want to seek out someone with a specialty in breast-feeding medicine (contact the Academy of Breastfeeding Medicine, https://www.abm.org). I want you to get the care you need quickly. You may be able to see a practitioner via Zoom if there is no one in your community.

CONCLUSION

Breast and nipple pain are frequent among breastfeeding mothers. Fortunately, in most cases, we can help you identify possible causes for your pain and take steps to address it. Don't believe it when you're told that everything is "fine" or that there's nothing you can do. You have many options. I want you to get relief as quickly as possible.

III

MILK PRODUCTION: HOW IT WORKS AND HOW TO SPOT DIFFICULTIES

INTRODUCTION: MILK PRODUCTION: HOW IT WORKS AND HOW TO SPOT DIFFICULTIES

New mothers often worry about having enough milk (DiTomasso et al., 2022). Perception of low supply is one of the most common reasons why mothers stop breastfeeding. In this section, I discuss how your body makes milk and how you can know, with confidence, that you're making enough. I'll describe what you need to look for and if your supply is low, how to increase it.

CHAPTER 7

MAKING MILK: HOW YOU CAN KNOW YOUR BABY IS GETTING ENOUGH

HOW YOUR BODY MAKES MILK

Your body is amazing. Not only did you create a tiny human, but you're also making the substance that keeps that human alive. Making and delivering milk involves a complex network of hormones, but the two key ones are oxytocin and prolactin. Prolactin makes the milk, and oxytocin releases it through the milk-ejection reflex (MER). Removing milk from the breast is the key; when milk is removed from your breasts, via baby or pump, your body makes more. You need to remove it eight to 12 times a day to establish and maintain a supply.

Milk production operates on supply and demand. The more your baby needs or "demands," the more your body makes. When your baby needs less, such as when they are starting solids, your body will slow supply. Your body will also ramp up supply at times, such as a growth spurt, when your baby needs more. People also use the factory as an illustration of this principle. When a lot of product is leaving the factory, the assembly line in your breasts makes sure that there is enough available. However, when you empty your breasts less often, product builds in the warehouse, and your factory supervisor tells your workers to slow down.

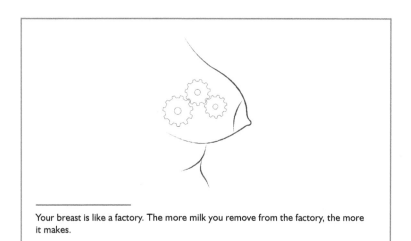

Your breast is like a factory. The more milk you remove from the factory, the more it makes.

If you don't remove milk, it backs up, and the immediate danger is mastitis. Mastitis is a hot, red area on your breast that can become infected. If you develop mastitis, keep feeding on that side. You can also use heat and gentle massage to move milk out of your breast. If you develop a fever or flulike symptoms, call your provider because you may have developed an infection. The secondary danger of not removing milk is that it tells your body to slow production through a hormone called FIL, or feedback inhibitor of lactation. If FIL is hanging around, your body continues to slow down milk production.

SETTING YOUR MILK PRODUCTION FOR THIS PREGNANCY

We used to think how much you fed in the first few days didn't matter in terms of setting mother's supply. Mothers were separated from their babies and providers introduced early bottles, even when not medically necessary. We were optimistic that mothers' supply could recover, but we now know that the first couple of weeks matter a lot. Early breastfeeding sets a cap for your milk production. Without frequent milk removals in the first 2 weeks, you may not have a full supply *for this pregnancy* (Mohrbacher & Kendall-Tackett, 2010). What this means is that if you're having a problem with milk supply now, it doesn't mean that you will have the same problem with another baby.

If possible, feed your baby right after birth before your baby has a long first sleep. After your baby wakes from their nap, hold them as much as you want. You cannot spoil your baby by doing this, and it's a great way to keep your baby calm. The first couple of weeks are all about transitioning your baby from womb to world (Colson, 2019). Postpartum doula Salle Webber made a similar observation in *The Gentle Art of Newborn Family Care* (Webber, 2012):

> The baby at this is time is transitioning between worlds. He needs human touch, voices, and the stimulation of skin-to-skin contact to remind him of his new place in life. We must draw him into worldly existence with our attention, love, and enthusiasm for his presence among us. (p. 20)

FREQUENT FEEDINGS

Your baby will have short, frequent feeds where they get an early milk called colostrum. Colostrum is super-concentrated milk that is loaded with antibodies to protect your baby from pathogens, coat their gut, and help them eliminate meconium.

Your feeding patterns are completely different from those of formula-feeding mothers, so you can't compare yourself with them. Those babies seem to feed less often and have to be on a schedule because adults need to control the amount they eat. It's quite easy to overfeed with a bottle because the flow is constant, and babies don't have to work to get milk out. That's the reason for the schedule.

In comparison, the pattern for breastfeeding can seem really erratic, and that can trip you up in the beginning. Current breastfeeding guidelines are that you should feed your baby eight to 12 times a day. When we hear that, we think that babies will eat every 2 to 3 hours. Unfortunately, babies haven't read the books. They may feed every hour for a while and then go longer stretches, and that would be within the normal range.

If you try to compare yourself with a formula-feeding mother, with their nice, orderly schedule, you'll be convinced you are doing it wrong. You aren't. Although I generally think you don't need to track everything (like minutes on each side), in the beginning, you may want to track the number of times you feed just to make sure you're feeding at least eight times a day. You can just make a tick on a piece of paper or whiteboard.

As a new mother, you'll quickly find that family, friends, and even strangers feel compelled to comment on how often your baby eats. If you're worried about it, check in with your baby's practitioner. As your baby matures, the feeding pattern will seem less erratic and will settle into a more regular rhythm.

The Role of Storage Capacity

Breast storage capacity refers to the amount of milk-making tissue you have in your breasts (Mohrbacher & Kendall-Tackett, 2010). Understanding the role of storage capacity can help you understand why your baby feeds the way they do and why your experience is unique. Storage capacity is not based on breast size. Mothers with small breasts may have loads of milk-making tissue. Conversely, mothers with large breasts may have little or a lot. Here's why this is relevant to feeding pattern.

Storage Capacity Dictates Feeding Pattern

Storage capacity influences how often you feed, how long each feeding lasts, whether you use one breast or two, and whether night feedings continue. So pretty much everything about your and your baby's feeding pattern. A mother with a large storage capacity may have fewer or shorter feedings, her baby may sleep longer stretches earlier, and her baby always takes one breast. Conversely, a mother with a small storage capacity may have more feedings over the day. The feedings may take longer, night feedings continue to be necessary, and her baby always uses both breasts. Over 24 hours, both mothers feed their babies the same amount of milk, but the pattern differs. Your baby will get all the milk they need if you follow their lead and feed when they indicate that it's time.

Because every mother–baby pair is unique, it makes no sense to compare yourself with others or to try to be "average." The woman who tells you that her baby is already sleeping longer at night may have a larger storage capacity. It has nothing to do with her skill as a mother. It's a quirk of her biology, like having blue eyes. You have no control over that, and neither does she. Don't go down that rabbit hole with her; it will make you worry about nothing.

When Milk Becomes More Abundant: Lactogenesis II

Around Day 3 to 4, your milk changes from colostrum to mature milk and becomes more abundant. We used to say that your milk has "come in," but that was a misnomer. Milk has been there all along, even during your pregnancy. During lactogenesis II (LG II), the composition of your milk has changed, and volume increases. Many mothers become engorged during this time, but frequent feeding reduces risk.

HOW CAN I TELL IF MY BABY IS GETTING ENOUGH TO EAT?

All new mothers want to know this. Honestly, it's one of the appeals of bottle-feeding: breastfeeding can seem like a bit of a black box. In the early days, it would be reassuring if breasts had measuring lines like a bottle.

Baby's Weight: The Gold Standard

If your baby is getting enough to eat, they will gain weight. All babies lose some weight after birth but will usually start gaining it back right away. We like to see a baby back to their birthweight by 2 weeks at the latest, and the minimal acceptable weight gain is 5 ounces (140 g) per week. Your baby's weight is an important barometer of how they are doing, but there are a few qualifiers and things to know about weight.

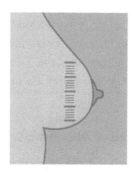

It would be handy if breasts had measuring lines so you could know how much your baby was getting.

What Do You Mean by Birthweight?

Birthweight is measured right after a baby is born. That seems logical, but what if you received a lot of fluids during your labor? If you did, your baby did too. Over the first 24 hours, they pee a lot to rid themselves of this extra fluid. Unfortunately, it looks like they've had a dramatic weight loss. Losing 7% of birthweight is cause for concern, but 10% or more can make hospital folk worry a lot, and they start pushing formula, as this mother describes:

> My son was breech, hence the planned cesarean. By Day 4, he had lost 11%, although every lactation consultant told me all looked good. On discharge day, the pediatrician came in to examine him, said "Mija, you're starving your baby," and handed me a can of formula.

The 24-Hour Birthweight Standard

In some cases, formula supplementation is the right move. However, what if the weight loss was actually only fluid that the baby picked up during birth, which they pee out in the first day of life? Is that actually a problem or does it just look like one? Researchers have examined birthweight and have determined that the 24-hour weight is a better predictor of problems with fewer false positives. By 24 hours, babies have peed out excessive fluid and hospitals got a truer sense of their actual weight. When hospitals have implemented the 24-hour birthweight standard, they supplemented less with no increase in adverse outcomes (Walker, 2018).

> The midwives and HCAs did try to support me with breast-feeding. In hindsight some was not great advice. I also had to do formula top-ups due to 12.5% weight loss. I wasn't told that they even had human milk at the hospital we could have used. And now looking back I expect the weight loss was due to fluids administered during a long and difficult labour.

An Accurate Weight

Some mothers feel better if they weigh their babies frequently. If that makes you feel less anxious, there's no harm in it. However, be consistent. It's kind of like when you weigh yourself. You need to make sure that the other variables stay the same so that you can tell if there was a small change.

- *Same scale*: Not all scales are calibrated the same, so you can weigh the same thing and get different weights. Scales can easily be off by a few ounces. Normally, that's not a huge problem, but if you are trying to detect small changes in your baby's weight, a few ounces can give you a completely false picture.
- *Good scale*: Consumer scales don't have the precision you need. Most pediatric, lactation, or well-baby clinics have scales you can use. These are more accurate.
- *Same state of dress*: Weigh your baby in just a diaper so you aren't looking for differences based on clothing. Also, don't weigh your baby with a wet diaper because next time it will look like they have lost weight when they haven't.

Poopy Diapers: The Yellow Standard

You can learn a lot from the number of poops and their delightful color.

Number of Daily Poops

Poop indicates that your baby is getting enough to eat. If your baby isn't pooping, they may not be getting enough to eat. Here's how many diapers you should be looking for. You are looking for a poop that is at least the size of a U.S. quarter, and anything smaller shouldn't be included in your count.

By Day 5, we want to see at least three to four poops at least the size of a U.S. quarter a day (.955 inch or 24.26 mm). If they are not pooping this much, don't panic, but do touch base with your provider to see if their weight gain is on track (Mohrbacher & Kendall-Tackett, 2010; Walker, 2018).

POOP COLOR

Your baby needs colostrum to help clear meconium from their gut, the black, tarry-looking poop. If meconium stays too long, your baby gets jaundice. As your milk becomes more abundant, your baby's poop will go from black to green to yellow. By about Day 4, your baby's poop should have transitioned to yellow. If it hasn't, don't panic, but don't ignore it either. Get your baby evaluated to make sure things are going well.

What about wet diapers? Wet diapers show that your baby is getting enough to drink and is not dehydrated. If you don't see wet diapers, touch base with your provider. Do you need to count wet diapers? You can if you want. By Day 3, the number will increase to four to six a day. If your baby is eating enough, they are most likely drinking enough too.

FALSE SIGNS THAT YOU DON'T HAVE ENOUGH MILK

For much of my career, I've worked with mothers who had ample supplies but were worried. I reassured them that everything was going well and told them why I thought that. In retrospect, I wish I would have also asked them why they were concerned. If you're worried, it's okay to ask for help or reassurance. The following are some common concerns that providers should evaluate but don't necessarily mean insufficient milk.

My Baby Is on the Breast "All the Time"

A baby taking a long time to feed does not necessarily mean that there is a problem, but it does warrant a closer look. Your baby may have trouble drinking milk, so we should try to figure out why. Or you may have a smaller storage capacity, which is not a problem, but it does mean more frequent feeds. If your baby is gaining weight but you feel like your baby is on "all the time," you might feel overwhelmed by the 24/7 nature of postpartum and need a short break. Feed your baby, let someone else hold them, and take a short break. The intensity eases up once your baby gets past the first few weeks.

My Baby Feeds More Often Than My Friend's

This could also be an issue of storage capacity: You may have less than your friend. Remember, you and your baby are unique. You can't compare your experience to anyone else's. Your pattern is the right one for you, and your baby is still getting the same amount of milk over a 24-hour period, but the pattern of delivery is probably different.

I Don't Get Anything When I Pump

Some people will suggest that if you want to know how much milk you are making, pump it out and you can see. If you easily let down to a pump, this could work for you. However, a lot of mothers need to practice with a pump, and the first few times they try, they get nothing. There are even a small number of mothers with full supplies who are never able to pump. Pumping tells them nothing about their supply. The type of pump also makes a difference. A lot of women have trouble with cheap pumps. If you need to pump a lot, such as when you return to work, you need a double-electric pump to maintain your supply. Finally, if you use the wrong setting on a pump, especially if it hurts, you won't get let down. Your baby is always going to be more efficient in removing milk than even the best pump. Bottom-line: Pumping is not a good indication of your milk supply. If your baby is gaining well, don't worry if there's nothing in the pump. Your baby is getting enough to eat.

My Baby Eats When I Give Them a Bottle

Because of the constant flow, babies eat more with a bottle. What does that mean? If you feed your baby at the breast and then give a top up with a couple of ounces in a bottle, it doesn't mean they were hungry. Babies will eat from bottles because the food is *there*, and they don't have to do anything to get it. It's like Doritos; you don't usually eat those because you are hungry but because they are crunchy, delicious, and come in Cool Ranch flavor—and because they are *there*. Babies are no different. How can you tell the difference between a hungry baby versus a baby eating Girl Scout cookies? Your baby's weight is the best indicator. Has their weight gain slowed, or are they losing weight? If your baby is actually hungry, there will be other signs besides just snarfing up what's in a bottle, such as excessive sleepiness or crying.

If you're concerned, get a weight check. And watch out for recommendations to give your baby a top-up with a bottle "just to be safe." You can't overfeed a baby at the breast, but adding top-ups they don't need will certainly result in overfeeding, which will make your baby miserable and possibly cause overeating as they get older (Li et al., 2010).

There's potentially one other problem with a top-off. If they become a regular part of your routine, your baby will remove less milk from your breast at their next feed. If feedings start getting spaced too far apart, your milk supply will suffer, and then formula will become necessary to make up the shortfall. It's the classic slippery slope.

CONCLUSION

You can feed your baby with confidence. Involve your partner or your support person. Know the signs of when your baby is getting enough to eat and don't feel like you need to go through this alone. Remove milk from your breasts at least eight times a day, make sure that your baby is pooping, and if in doubt, have your baby weighed on the same scale.

CHAPTER 8

DELAYED LACTOGENESIS II AND INSUFFICIENT MILK SUPPLY

In some situations where breastfeeding did not work and babies were harmed, mothers had reached out to providers who ignored signs or didn't know what to look for. They thought that they were "supporting breastfeeding" by telling mothers to "keep doing what you're doing" without doing a proper assessment. Supporting breastfeeding doesn't mean ignoring problems and sticking your head in the sand. Instead, problems need to be identified and addressed quickly. The focus of this chapter is what to look for and what to do when there is a real problem with milk supply. In most cases, it's possible to avert a crisis and get breastfeeding back on track.

SIGNS OF DEHYDRATION: GET HELP RIGHT AWAY

Master lactation consultant Marsha Walker compiled the following list of red flags for parents. She recommended that parents "trust your instincts. Get help right away if something doesn't seem right" (Walker, 2018; p. 181).

- Your baby does not have a wet diaper for longer than 6 hours. If you're using disposable diapers, it will feel heavier if it's wet or some brands change colors.
- Urine is dark and smells strong.

- Your baby is lethargic, limp, or docile.
- Your baby has a dry mouth.
- Your baby is irritable. Babies can be irritable for many reasons—even if they are well-fed but check milk supply first.
- Your baby has inconsolable crying. Crying can also be a sign of hunger. Beyond hunger, it could be sensitive temperament, exposure to too many people, or a possible injury at birth.
- Your baby has a sunken fontanel (the soft spot on the top of their head), a fever, skin with a yellow tinge, or skin that tents when it's pinched up.

Source: Marsha Walker (2018). Used with permission.

DELAYED LACTOGENESIS II

For most women, lactogenesis II (LG II), when milk becomes more abundant, happens by Day 3 or 4. However, it can also be delayed. This is why mothers and babies need to be evaluated at 72 to 96 hours postpartum (Dewey et al., 2003; Walker, 2018). Although 72 to 96 hours postpartum is the guideline, few American women are evaluated this early. The standard from the American Academy of Pediatrics is a visit by 48 to 72 hours after discharge or 3 to 5 days after birth (Taylor & Parekh, 2020).

Walker lists risk factors for delayed LG II. They don't mean that you won't be able to breastfeed, but you will need some support. Use the strategies in the next section to jumpstart LG II.

Mother's Risk Factors

Some mothers are more at risk for delayed LG II.

- *First-time mother.* First-time mothers worry more about their milk supplies and are more likely to supplement (DiTomasso et al., 2022).

- *Stressful, traumatic, or surgical delivery.* High levels of the stress hormone cortisol suppress prolactin, the hormone that makes milk (Grajeda & Pérez-Escamilla, 2002).
- *History of low milk supply.* You may be fine this time, but let's check.
- *Diabetes.* Excess insulin can block prolactin.
- *Polycystic ovary syndrome (PCOS)* is another condition in which insulin levels can be too high.
- *Hypothyroidism.* Low thyroid can also be a factor in insufficient milk supply. If you take thyroid replacement, this usually isn't a problem. However, some mothers, particularly those with gestational diabetes, develop hypothyroidism in the postpartum period (Kendall-Tackett, 2017).
- *Significant hemorrhage or retained placental fragment.* Although it's fairly rare, a significant hemorrhage can delay LG II or cause insufficient milk supply. Similarly, a placental fragment left behind in your uterus blocks prolactin and may need to be surgically removed before breastfeeding can commence.
- *Sore nipples.* The most common cause of sore nipples is a shallow latch, which makes feeding painful for the mother but can also mean that the baby is not transferring milk out of the breast, which can lead to delayed LG II and possible low supply.

Baby's Risk Factors

Your baby may also have risk factors that contribute to delayed LG II.

- *Preterm or late preterm.* Neonatal intensive care units have made great strides in helping mothers of preterm infants protect their supply and transition to feeding at the breast. But sometimes they don't, and LG II can be delayed. Late preterm babies, born at 34 to 36 weeks' gestation, are trickier. Marsha Walker called them the "little imposters" because they look like full-term infants, but they are not (Walker, 2020). These babies are at high risk for rehospitalization for jaundice or dehydration. They fall asleep at the breast before they get a full feed, which wears mothers out and can compromise their supply.

Make sure your baby is not too warm because that can make them sleepy. Massage the soles of their feet and use breast compression when their suckling slows. In some cases, you might need to pump and feed your baby your expressed milk from a bottle or supplementary nursing system. As they eat more, they can stay awake longer. This is true for all babies, but preterm and late preterm babies may be particularly susceptible.

- *Small or large for gestational age.* This can also influence their sleepiness and their effectiveness in draining your breast.
- *Delivered via forceps or vacuum extraction.* Your baby's skull bones are malleable so that they can fit down the birth canal. A vacuum extraction or forceps, or any vaginal birth, may subtly move the bones of your baby's skull. An infant chiropractor or craniosacral therapist can gently realign the bones and make things more comfortable for them (Berg-Drazin, 2019; Lavigne, 2016; Miller, 2019, 2020).
- *Loss of more than 7% of their birthweight.* Excessive weight loss can be a concern, but before you panic, read the discussion in the previous chapter about using the 24-hour birthweight.
- *No audible swallowing.* If you do not hear swallowing, your baby is not drinking milk.
- *Multiple births.* Even when you have more than one baby, you can make enough milk, but you will need lots of support. Your babies may have been early, in the NICU, or both. You may have one at home and the others still at the hospital.

Some Signs of Delayed LG II You Might Observe in Your Baby

- *Jaundice.* With jaundice, your baby's skin has a yellow tinge—your provider will probably prescribe time under a Bili-light, which eliminates bilirubin in their blood so that they can pass it out of their systems. They may also suggest that you feed more frequently to increase the amount of breast milk that your baby is receiving to help them pass bilirubin.
- *Crying and never satisfied.* Hunger is one cause of crying, so we need to investigate that first. Crying can also be due to temperament, too many people around, or a birth injury. Infant chiropractor Dr. Joyce Miller has had great success with lessening inconsolable crying through gentle chiropractic and has demonstrated its efficacy in controlled trials (Miller, 2019, 2020).
- *Takes longer than 30 minutes to feed.* If it seems like it takes your baby a long time to eat, have someone take a look. There could be an issue, or you may have a small storage capacity and it's a normal pattern for you.
- *Extreme sleepiness.* New parents are often thrilled when their baby sleeps a lot, but make sure that they are not sleeping through mealtimes.

Strategies for Delayed LG II

If you have a delay in LG II, Marsha Walker (2018) suggested some things that can help.

- *Breast massage and the milk shake.* Gently shaking your breast and doing gentle massage before you put your baby on.
- *Empty your breasts a minimum of 10 times a day via your baby or a pump.* You will need to empty your breasts more often than mothers whose LG II is not delayed. You might try

adding a pumping session a couple of times a day (after the first-morning feed is often a good time).

- *Feed your baby during light sleep.* Watch for REM (rapid eye movement) sleep, where you'll see your baby's eyes move under their lids—feeding while in light sleep also works well with babies who refuse the breast. They are more willing while they are sleeping.

- *If you need to supplement, use your milk, donor milk, or hypoallergenic formula.* Marsha Walker (2018) suggested hypoallergenic formula because it is less likely to affect your baby's gut microbiome than regular formula. Standard formulas contain whole proteins that can cause imbalances in gut bacteria, which can lead to allergies. In contrast, hypoallergenic formulas do not include whole proteins but instead include basic amino acids (the building blocks of proteins), and these are least likely to cause allergic reactions.

SUPPLEMENTING AT-BREAST FEEDING

In addition to feeding at the breast, you may need to supplement at-breast feeding using a cup, feeding syringe, dropper, spoon, supplementary nursing system, or bottle. The amount your baby needs per feed is listed below. If you pump or hand express and it seems like you can only express a little bit, don't worry. It takes practice to get the hang of a pump, and your volume will increase after LG II.

- Day 1: 2–10 mL (1–2 teaspoons)/feed
- First 24 hours: 5–15 mL (1–3 teaspoons)/feed
- Days 2–3: 15–30 mL (3 teaspoons to 1 oz)/feed
- Days 4–5: 30–60 mL (1–2 oz)/feed

Source: Marsha Walker (2018). Used with permission.

INSUFFICIENT MILK

Insufficient milk production means that mothers do not make enough milk to fully feed their babies. Insufficient milk may be temporary or, in some cases, permanent. Many of the risk factors associated with delayed LG II can also contribute to insufficient milk, but they are not the same thing. Some common causes are the following.

Too Few Milk Removals

When a mother is concerned about her supply, I first ask how many times a day is she emptying her breasts. If the number is less than eight, we start by increasing the number of milk removals. Many times we can get things back on track. Spacing or timing feedings can lower the number of milk removals. The same can be true for pacifiers. I've never held the view that pacifiers are "the devil's teat," but they can space out feedings, which, before you know it, can drop your supply. If you decide to use one, wait until at least 4 weeks to introduce it (American Academy of Pediatrics, 2016).

Dropped Night Feedings or When You Return to Work

You may have had a full supply only to see it drop once you thought it was established. One common cause is dropped nighttime feeding when your baby starts sleeping through the night. A lowered supply can also happen with work or when you're on holiday as the number of pumping sessions or times you nurse your baby drops. If it hasn't been too long since you noticed a dip, you should be able to bring your production back up.

Medications

Some medications cause milk production to plummet. Birth control pills are a common culprit, especially if they have estrogen. Even progestin-only birth control pills can cause problems for some mothers. Wait at least 6 weeks before using any type of oral or hormonal contraceptives.

Antihistamines like Sudafed are also notorious for causing lower supply. Cold medications can have a similar effect if they have an antihistamine. Pay attention to any medication you take to see whether it influences your milk production. If you see a dip, find an alternative if possible.

Herbs and Botanicals

Some botanicals can block milk production. Two of the big culprits are peppermint and sage (Marasco & West, 2019). Mothers may take these having no idea that they can cause a problem. These two herbs have such a strong effect that we sometimes give them to mothers who are making too much milk and want to rein in their supply.

Placenta Encapsulation

If you're worried about supply, I'd steer clear of placenta encapsulation (PE). I know many in the breastfeeding community who swear by PE, and you may argue with me about this, but there are some concerns that I hope you will at least weigh. PE is when a mother has her placenta dried, ground, and put in capsules. Part of the rationale for this practice is that animals do it in the wild (to protect their babies from predators). The idea is that if animals do it, it is good for humans too. However, animals eat theirs raw, so the argument doesn't really follow.

The other rationale for PE is that it replaces hormones that are lost during birth. I've known for many years about this practice and the claims for its many positive benefits. For years, it was a very fringe practice, and then it started being more mainstream. Many mothers have said it made all the difference for them. They didn't get depressed, and they had tons of milk. As more women were doing it, people started raising concerns. In 2017, the U.S. Centers for Disease Control and Prevention urged caution with PE because of possible strep contamination that infected a baby (Buser et al., 2017).

Bacterial contamination is one concern. I'd also like to address the issue of efficacy. PE has been marketed as a way to prevent postpartum depression, with the rationale being that it replaces lost estrogen. Unfortunately, the rationale behind PE—to replace lost estrogen—was based on an old and refuted theory of postpartum depression. Postpartum depression is not caused by a drop in estrogen and progesterone (Kendall-Tackett, 2017). Not surprisingly, no proper randomized trial has found that PE lowers the risk of depression.

To demonstrate that it actually works, you would need a double-blind trial, as you would need this research design to test the efficacy of any substance, including medications. To do a study like this, someone would need to make capsules with placentas and make similar-looking capsules made of something else (like steak). Neither the mothers nor the investigators handing out the capsules would know which one the mother was receiving (that's why it's called a "double-blind" study because neither the participants nor investigators know who is in the treatment group). At the end of the study, you measure the variable you are interested in, like depression, to see if it really worked. This design is necessary to account for the placebo effect. Our minds are powerful. If you think something will work, it very well may, even if it's an inert substance. We have no study like this, even though it wouldn't be hard to do. Lately, proponents have said that it's not estrogen that works, but that PE replaces iron. Iron replacement can be a good thing if someone is anemic. However, there are cheaper, safer, and tastier ways to do that.

If people were only using PE for preventing depression, I'd probably not say anything. However, another concern is what PE can do to milk supply (Cole, 2014). Oddly, for the past few years, PE has been marketed as a way to *increase* your milk supply, which makes no sense physiologically. Estrogen stays in your placental tissue. When you eat or take your placenta as a capsule, you are taking estrogen. In Sonoma County, California, the lactation consultants started tracking mothers who could not bring in a full milk supply. They discovered that all of these mothers had used PE (Hollister, 2018). The Sonoma County Breastfeeding Coalition has put together a website called "Placenta Risks." It goes into a lot more detail, and if you are considering PE, you might want to check it out.

BREAST INJURY OR BREAST SURGERY

Breast surgery of any kind, including augmentation or reduction, can cause a problem with milk supply, but it doesn't always. Breast surgery is less likely to interfere if the nerves are intact, especially around the areola. But sometimes injury comes from unexpected sources. A mother I worked with could not establish a full supply with one of her breasts. It turns out that when she was a tiny preterm baby, she had a chest tube, which damaged her intercostal nerve and made it impossible to breastfeed on that side.

When mothers have had a breast reduction, another key question is whether the surgeon injured or removed milk ducts. If they did, full breastfeeding might not be possible. That being said, I've known mothers who had incredibly invasive surgeries, where there is no physical way they should be breastfeeding, yet they establish a full supply. Don't give up hope but be realistic and vigilant. I'd encourage you to read Diana West's (2001) book, *Defining Your Own Success.* She is the expert on the effects of breast surgery, and she provides many helpful suggestions.

INSUFFICIENT GLANDULAR TISSUE

Insufficient glandular tissue (IGT) is when mothers do not have enough milk-making tissue to bring in a full supply. These mothers often work incredibly hard trying to breastfeed, but it doesn't work the way they planned. Although there are many case studies and personal stories in the literature about IGT, there is much we do not know. The incidence and causes are unknown. It appears to be fairly rare, but it does occur. If you read the information that follows and suspect that you have IGT, work closely with a provider so that they can spot any feeding issues early and give you alternative strategies for feeding your baby (Cassar-Uhl, 2014).

There are a few telltale symptoms of IGT, including breasts of markedly different sizes, tubular breasts, or a hand's-width space between your breasts. If you had surgery, it might have been to cover up these symptoms and change the appearance of your breasts. If you think this might apply to you, think back to what your breasts looked like before your surgery.

Mothers with IGT often experience grief, shame, and loss when they are unable to breastfeed. If you think you might have IGT, please know that you didn't cause this. Breastfeeding is still possible, but it is unlikely to be a full supply. You can pump and supply your milk, but please be easy on yourself with regard to difficult pumping regimens. While it's great that your baby is getting your milk, that shouldn't come at the cost of your mental health. Your relationship with your baby and mental health must take priority here. I'd suggest using the strategies I describe in Chapter 18 and also checking out Diana Cassar-Uhl's (2014) book, *Finding Sufficiency.*

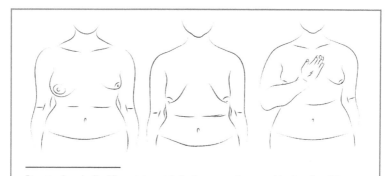

Breasts of markedly different sizes, tubular breasts, or breasts with a hand's width between them can be symptoms of insufficient glandular tissue (IGT).

BABIES WHO ARE SLEEPY AT THE BREAST

Babies who are sleepy at the breast can compromise your milk production because they don't drain your breasts thoroughly. Some of these babies are late preterm. They could have jaundice or labor medications could make them sleepy. They may also be overdressed, which makes them too warm. These babies can also be sensitive. Sometimes a loud or chaotic environment can cause them to shut down rather than sleep, which could lead to missed feedings. Many late preterm babies tire easily, and their feeding patterns can wear you out because they often fall asleep before they get enough to eat. At the breast, they are suck-suck-suck-sleep and then are back 20 minutes later with the same pattern. The challenge here is to get enough calories into them before they conk out.

Here is a hack that might help. It also helps when you pump. Our goal is to release the fattier milk in your milk ducts so that it is available to your baby more quickly. Fattier milk may keep them satisfied a bit longer and make sure that they are well-fed. There are two steps: massage and the "milk shake," and breast compressions.

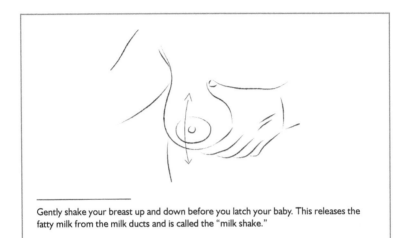

Gently shake your breast up and down before you latch your baby. This releases the fatty milk from the milk ducts and is called the "milk shake."

Massage and Milk Shake

A video demonstration of the milk shake and breast compressions.

Gently massage, stroking your breasts toward your nipple. While you are doing that, gently shake your breasts before you feed your baby. Both of these activities release fat into your milk. Be very gentle. This should not hurt.

Breast Compressions

After you have massaged and shaken your breasts, feed normally. When suckling slows or your baby looks drowsy, gently compress your breast. Use your fingers and thumb in a C position and gently squeeze. Your baby should start sucking again in earnest. The keyword here is *gentle*. If it hurts, it's too hard.

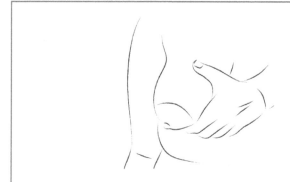

Gentle compressions of your breast also keep the milk flowing and release the fattier milk. Gently squeeze and hold. When your baby slows down, find another place on your breast and gently compress and hold.

When suckling slows again, move your fingers to another part of your breast and squeeze. Suckling should increase as the milk flow increases. This technique also helps get more milk flowing when you pump. It can help if you have a plugged duct because it helps release milk from different places on your breast when you do a gentle compression. In the meantime, if your baby has a lot of clothing on, try taking some of it off to see if that helps wake them up.

STRATEGIES

There are some things you can do to increase your supply, but some of these strategies can be difficult and overwhelming. Use your best judgment. If the strategies are short term and not too onerous, they are worth trying. However, I've met many mothers who exhaust themselves with rigorous regimens. Only you can decide whether a regimen is worth it, but I'd encourage you to also consider the options I describe in Chapter 18. Breastfeeding is important, but so is your well-being and your relationship with your baby.

Increase Milk Removals (to a Point)

Some lactation consultants tell mothers to pump every 2 hours around the clock to protect or boost their supply. Don't do that! That routine will trash your mental health in no time. Don't set an alarm. You'll naturally wake when your breasts are full. If you wake naturally, you'll be less fatigued because you'll wake at a better time in terms of your sleep cycles. If your baby is also awake, go ahead and feed them.

Have your pump and a cooler to put your milk in near your bed. Use a low light so that you don't completely wake up. Don't worry about cleaning your pump in between your nighttime pumping sessions. Breastmilk has active white blood cells that keep bacteria in check so it will be okay until morning. Clean it then and put your milk in the refrigerator.

Cluster Pump

For mothers with a low supply, New York City lactation consultant Catherine Watson Genna suggested a strategy called cluster pumping. For a short period of time, pump every hour. Cathy suggests that you set your pump in a high-traffic area of your home and have a 10- to 15-minute pumping session every time you walk by. You can, say, pump every hour for 4 hours. There are many variations of this strategy. She suggests that you have some chocolates (or something else you'd enjoy) by your pump. If you need four extra sessions, set out four candies. Every time you pump, you get one. It's an easy and enjoyable way to keep track of your extra sessions. This is meant to be a temporary strategy, not long term.

GALACTAGOGUES: THINGS YOU CAN TAKE TO BOOST SUPPLY

Before you use a galactagogue, make sure that the basics are in place, including the number of milk removals and an effective latch. Second, some of these products interact with prescription medications and could potentially endanger your health, so check with your health care provider before you take any of them. This is only a partial list of herbs purported to boost supply. Some have long histories as folk remedies, but don't, necessarily, have evidence that supports their use. If you want to know your full range of options, I'd encourage you to read Lisa Marasco and Diana West's (2019) book, *Making More Milk*.

Fenugreek and Blessed Thistle

Fenugreek and blessed thistle are the best known of herbal galactagogues, which have a long folk history of use but not a lot of evidence to support their use. Food manufacturers make imitation maple syrup from fenugreek, so one side effect you might experience is urine and sweat that smells like maple syrup. Although fenugreek is generally safe, there have been some interactions with prescription medications, and it lowers blood sugar in people with diabetes (Ruddle, 2021). Some women are allergic to it (especially if they have a legume or peanut allergy), so talk it over with your provider to see if fenugreek would be safe for you (Newman, n.d.-b).

Dr. Jack Newman (n.d.-b) recommended three capsules three times a day for both fenugreek and blessed thistle. If your milk supply doesn't increase, you can increase the dose to four capsules three times a day of each.

Goat's Rue

Goat's rue is another herb that comes from the same family as fenugreek. Goat's rue contains a constituent that can be used to create the medication metformin (used for Type 2 diabetes and PCOS). For this reason, it may be particularly helpful for women who have a low supply due to PCOS. The dose is 20 to 40 drops three times a day (Newman, n.d.-b).

Shatavari

Shatavari is a substance used in Ayurvedic medicine and is from the same family as asparagus. It, too, can lower blood sugar levels, so close monitoring is important for women with diabetes. Its traditional use is for infertility and increasing milk supply. The dose is one to two 500-mg capsules two times a day (Newman, n.d.-b).

Moringa

Moringa, another plant-based galactagogue, is from the Philippines. There is some evidence for its effectiveness. In one randomized trial with mothers of preterm infants, it increased supply (Estrella et al., 2000). Take three to four times a day, up to 4.5 grams (Newman, n.d.-b). Moringa can also lower blood sugar, so monitor your levels more frequently if you have diabetes.

TINCTURES AND TEAS

Traditional Medicinal makes tea for nursing mothers, and MotherLove herbal makes teas, tinctures, and capsules using a variety of herbs. Many mothers find these products helpful. Teas often contain a combination of herbs, such as fennel, fenugreek, and blessed thistle. The dose from a tea will be substantially less than a capsule or tincture.

Some naturopaths may also suggest teas with calming herbs, such as lemon balm and chamomile.

Tinctures are compounds in which concentrated herbs are preserved in an alcohol base. You use a dropper to measure the dose. Tinctures may combine herbs, or they could be a single herb, such as fenugreek or blessed thistle. Again, there's an absence of double-blind trials. Most are safe, but let your health care provider know you are using them because they can influence blood sugar and may interact with other medications. Follow the manufacturer's instructions or use 20 drops three times a day (Newman, n.d.-b).

Galactagogue Foods

Foods such as oatmeal and brewer's yeast are purported to be galactagogues. There's no evidence that these foods make any difference. If you enjoy these foods, there's no harm in them, but don't make yourself eat foods you don't enjoy in order to try to boost your supply.

Beer is another purported galactagogue. It does not boost supply, but you can have one anyway. Nurse your baby first and then imbibe. It takes about 2 hours for a single drink to clear from your system and your milk (Hale, 2021).

Lactation Cookies

Lactation cookies are tasty, but again, there's no evidence that they boost supply. If you want a cookie, have one. Have two. If you want to whip up a batch of your own, there are loads of recipes online. Cost is my main concern with commercial lactation cookies. Some mothers feel that they must have these to breastfeed. It's not true. If you're worried about supply, make sure to empty your breasts at least 10 times a day and check in with a lactation consultant. If you need help with your milk supply, there are more effective ways to increase it than eating cookies.

Pharmaceutical Galactagogues

Two prescription medications increase milk supply: metoclopramide and domperidone. Both of these medications were used to increase gut motility in older patients (and help them have bowel movements) when people discovered a weird side effect—increased prolactin, which increases milk supply. Using these medications to boost milk supply is considered an off-label use.

In the United States, domperidone has been banned by the Food and Drug Administration because of possible cardiac arrhythmias. That is serious, but if you look at the studies, the dose of domperidone is much higher in the older patients than it would be for mothers wanting to increase milk supply. In addition, arrhythmias appeared in older men who were already ill (Hale et al., 2018).

Generally speaking, domperidone is far safer for mothers than the alternative: metoclopramide (Reglan). In our study of 1,880 mothers who had taken one or both medications as galactagogues, we asked them to report side effects. Cardiac side effects were rare (less than 1%) but were higher with metoclopramide than domperidone (Hale et al., 2018). From a mental health standpoint, I'd urge you to avoid Reglan (metoclopramide) if at all possible because it increased the risk of depression by 7 times in our study (Hale et al., 2018).

Getting domperidone in the United States is tricky. Some mothers nip over to Canada to buy it, and some order them from New Zealand or Vanuatu. You might not feel comfortable with that, and depending on where you live, it might be illegal. You might be able to get it from a compounding pharmacy, but some will not fill the prescription. One book that talks about how to use domperidone is Alyssa Schnell's *Breastfeeding Without Birthing* (Schnell, 2013). Domperidone can also be used to induce lactation in parents who have not given birth, and it is useful for birth mothers too. Her book gives detailed instructions on how to use it. Dr. Jack Newman's site

127

for the International Breastfeeding Centre also has information on how to use domperidone (https://www.ibconline.ca).

CONCLUSION

Concerns about delayed LG II and insufficient milk supply are relatively common and a frequent reason why mothers seek lactation care (DiTomasso et al., 2022). For most mothers, delayed LG II or insufficient milk supply can be addressed, and breastfeeding proceeds normally. For a smaller percentage of mothers, underlying conditions make it impossible to bring in a full supply. If that happens, you still have options and ways to feed and bond with your baby. I hope you will stay with me as I go into detail about these options in Chapter 18.

IV

SLEEP AND NIGHTTIME FEEDING

INTRODUCTION: SLEEP AND NIGHTTIME FEEDING

Sleep is the most salient issue you face as a new mother, and you may be so exhausted that you worry that breastfeeding will be a casualty. Some days, possibly even today, you might feel like you will die if you don't get some sleep. Lack of sleep can be one of the hardest things to cope with during the early days.

Being tired is common among new mothers, and most days, you can cope with it. But there is a difference between normal fatigue and complete exhaustion. I call it the difference between "tired" (normal) and "*more* tired" (not normal). More tired is much harder to cope with. In the early days, the siren song of formula draws you near with the promise of sleep. It's so tempting, but as with the sirens of legend, their song about sleep is an illusion. If you're skeptical, read on. Recent studies demonstrate that breastfeeding mothers actually get more sleep, which seems impossible, but it's true.

If you are exhausted and hanging on by a thread, this section can help. Skip to the end of Chapter 9 for strategies on what you can do to cope. You don't have to just tough it out.

CHAPTER 9

BREASTFEEDING, SLEEP, AND MENTAL HEALTH

Babies wake during the night because they need to. It's just the way they are made, but this can be so hard on new parents. It would be lovely for them to fit into our schedules and sleep all night, but they won't for a while. You may feel pressured to get your baby to sleep because everyone keeps asking you, "Is your baby sleeping through the night?"

People often have weird expectations about how much babies should sleep. They equate long stretches of sleep with being "good." That's nonsense, but it can make you wonder what you are doing wrong. Your baby is unique and that means a unique sleeping pattern. There is no "bad" or "good" here; there's just sleep.

It's not only normal for your baby to wake at night, it's healthy. Babies who wake frequently are less likely to die from sudden infant death syndrome (SIDS)—every parent's worst nightmare (Blair et al., 2020; McKenna, 2020). That's important but, in the middle of the night, it may not be comforting. Therefore, I want to help you cope with this (fortunately) brief time in your life.

HOW YOU FEED YOUR BABY DETERMINES
HOW MUCH SLEEP YOU GET

Everyone agrees that sleep is important for your mental health. Unfortunately, many providers do not understand how breastfeeding changes sleep. It is completely different, so much so that noted mother–baby sleep expert Dr. James McKenna invented a new term for it: *breastsleeping* (Blair et al., 2020).

When mental health providers make recommendations to new mothers about sleep, they often think in general terms but do not understand the fundamental relationship between feeding method and sleep. A few years ago, I was a guest for an online panel discussing mother–infant sleep. It was broadcast out of the United Kingdom and was the middle of the night for me, so I was a bit blurry. I could definitely empathize with the new mothers we were discussing, but even in my sleep-deprived state I needed to challenge the prevailing wisdom that some of my fellow panelists were presenting. A psychiatrist on the panel kept saying the mothers needed to sleep a set number of hours to protect their mental health. Every time he said this, I asked how the mothers were feeding. I was like a broken record. He thought it was irrelevant, yet it's one of the most important questions you can ask. Why? Because one type of feeding protects your mental health, the other does not.

Sleep for an Exclusively Breastfeeding Mother

For much of my career, I believed that breastfeeding mothers got less sleep. How could they not? They wake more, so they sleep less, right? What I couldn't figure out was why breastfeeding mothers had lower rates of depression. It was a real conundrum. I even put it in writing (Kendall-Tackett, 2007). Even in our study, the Survey of Mothers' Sleep and Fatigue, we found that exclusively breastfeeding mothers woke more and their babies had the shortest stretch of sleep (Kendall-Tackett et al., 2011). The first variable is mothers' report of how long their babies sleep at the longest stretch during the night. If mothers were exclusively breastfeeding (EBF), their infants slept 5.41 hours at the longest stretch compared with 7.69 hours for infants who were exclusively formula-fed (EFF).

When considering how babies are fed, our finding that EFF babies slept the longest time makes sense. Formula has foreign proteins that take longer to digest than breastmilk, so EBF babies wake sooner because their stomachs empty sooner, so their mothers report the shortest stretch. While that nice long stretch may seem nice for the mothers (at least on the surface), it's not great for the babies. According to Dr. James McKenna, anthropologist and foremost expert on mother–infant sleep, long stretches of infant sleep are risky (McKenna, 2020). A prominent theory of SIDS is that babies get into such a deep state of sleep that they are unable to rouse themselves. Nature designed a system of night waking to save babies, so sleeping a shorter time protects them. But what about you and your mental health? At first glance, it may seem like formula would protect your sleep too. Keep reading.

The plot thickens.

Let's look at another variable: the number of times that babies wake during the night. We see a similar pattern. The exclusively breastfed babies wake more times (2.52 times for EBF vs. 1.39 times for EFF). Again, that likely protects them from SIDS, but for a tired mom, that's not good news. In fact, it kind of sucks.

If you are only considering these data, I understand why mental health providers believe that mothers should not exclusively breastfeed. But that's not the whole picture.

More Sleep for Exclusively Breastfeeding Mothers

Three studies have found that the exclusively breastfeeding mothers get more sleep, even with more night wakings and shorter stretches of sleep. Theresa Doan and her colleagues (2007) were the first to study this, with a sample of 133 mothers. They found that exclusively breastfeeding mothers got about 20 minutes more sleep than mixed- or formula-feeding mothers. They also found that partners got more sleep if they fed the baby a bottle of breast milk versus formula. With their smaller sample size, you might think it was just a quirk of the data.

Dørheim et al.'s (2009a) sample included 2,831 mothers at 7 weeks postpartum. Not surprisingly, fatigue increased the risk of depression, but what were the factors associated with fatigue? They included being a first-time mom, having a baby who was an "early" or male infant, having a history of depression, and *not exclusively breastfeeding*. In other words, they found that *if you were mixed- or formula-feeding, you got less sleep, had more fatigue, and were more likely to be depressed.*

One of my editors wondered whether this finding was due to social class (with lower-income mothers getting less sleep) or having a live-in partner. It's an interesting question. Mothers with higher incomes may have been more likely to breastfeed because they have more access to resources that support them, so it could be their social class rather than their feeding method that made a difference here. Income wasn't included in the Dørheim study, so they couldn't check this as a competing theory. A live-in partner might also increase breastfeeding success.

I thought about the possible effect of income or having a live-in partner, recognizing that Dørheim's findings were the same as ours (see the next section). We did measure income in our U.S. contingent (4,789 mothers in our sample). Because we actively recruited from WIC programs, we had a large number of lower-income mothers in our sample. (WIC is a U.S. governmental supplemental feeding program for lower-income women, infants, and children.)

Across the whole sample, we had a full range of income levels, which essentially controlled for income. We had the same findings, so I do not believe that this finding was due to income. As for partner, 93% of our sample were living with a partner, and we still found a difference based on feeding method. We can't really attribute the findings to having a partner either.

SLEEP VARIABLES RELATED TO MATERNAL MENTAL HEALTH

The third study was ours. The first two variables I discuss are ones that sleep researchers have identified as relevant to mothers' mental health: their self-reported total sleep time and the number of minutes that it takes to get to sleep. We examined these variables with a sample of 6,410 mothers (Kendall-Tackett et al., 2011).

Mothers' Self-Reported Sleep Time

We also found that exclusively breastfeeding mothers slept an average of 20 to 30 minutes longer than other mothers (6.61 hours for EBF mothers vs. 6.3 for EFF mothers). In our post hoc analyses, we were shocked to discover *no significant difference between mixed- and formula-feeding on any of our variables*. Babies who are mixed-fed get the benefit of every ounce of breastmilk, and both mom and baby get all the lovely benefits of babies at the breast. However, our findings indicate that *for mothers*, only exclusive breastfeeding protects their sleep and, therefore, their mental health. We found this same pattern for every variable. On the basis of our findings, we concluded that *exclusive breastfeeding is a different physiological entity than other types of feeding*.

A more recent study surprisingly found this same pattern in the hospital, where no one is getting any sleep (Hughes et al., 2018). This study included 30 mothers in the first 48 hours postpartum and found that exclusively breastfeeding mothers slept 2.6 hours longer compared with mothers who were bottle-feeding. In the whole sample, mothers slept about 9.7 hours in the first 48 hours. That's not very much sleep, so 2.6 hours is significant. The authors concluded that exclusive breastfeeding promotes mothers' sleep. This is possibly an effect of oxytocin making it easier for mothers to sleep in the chaotic hospital environment.

Minutes to Get to Sleep

Another important sleep variable is the number of minutes it takes to get to sleep. Research is quite consistent on this. Twenty minutes or less is good and is associated with lower rates of depression. Twenty-five minutes or longer means that mothers are at higher risk for depression (Dørheim et al., 2009b; Goyal et al., 2007; Kendall-Tackett et al., 2011). In our findings, EBF mothers took 19.61 minutes to get to sleep compared with 27.05 for EFF mothers.

   Why might EBF help with sleep? Oxytocin is one possible explanation. Oxytocin opposes the stress response, and the stress response keeps you awake. With every milk let-down, you get a burst of oxytocin. When oxytocin is high, it relaxes you and helps you sleep. It's a remarkably coordinated system. Oxytocin is essential for milk ejection, and it increases during skin-to-skin contact. Snuggling in with your baby will make you tired, and you don't need to completely wake up to feed your baby.

   When mothers mixed- or formula-fed, someone has to get out of bed, turn on a light, and go to the kitchen to make up a bottle. Having a bottle by the bed helps if you need to bottle-feed, but you still need to wake up. Even if someone else is handling night feedings, chances are that you will hear the baby first because you are hormonally wired to be sensitive to your baby's cues. If there is a delay in getting the baby their meal, babies can be in quite a state. By the time you calm and feed the baby, everyone is wide awake, which can make it hard to fall asleep again.

HOW DOES THIS AFFECT MOTHERS?

You may be tempted to think, "That's such a small difference in total sleep time. I can't believe that that will affect my mental health." We asked mothers questions about their overall well-being. All of the things we asked lined up with our findings on the two key sleep variables. For example, when we asked them to rate their daily energy, no one is energetic during this time. On a 5-point scale, EBF mothers rated their daily energy as 3.01 versus 2.79 for EFF. It was slightly lower for mixed-feeding mothers. Given these findings, does it give mothers more energy when their babies got a bottle? The answer is clearly no.

Another measure of well-being is mothers' rating of their overall physical health. If you don't think of yourself as healthy, you are less likely to do things to keep yourself healthy. It's also related to confidence. If you don't think of yourself as healthy, do you believe that your body is capable of birthing a baby or sustaining them through breastfeeding? Consistent with our other findings, exclusively breast-feeding mothers were significantly more likely to rate their health as "very good" or "excellent." As I mentioned earlier, because we had a full range of incomes in the largest segment of our sample, I do not believe we can attribute this difference to social class.

DEPRESSIVE SYMPTOMS

The final variable is mothers' depressive symptoms. Consistent with Dørheim et al., we found lower depression for exclusively breast-feeding mothers with no significant difference between mixed- and formula-feeding. Depressive symptoms ranged from 0.85 for EBF mothers to 1.28 for EFF mothers.

On the basis of our findings and those of Dørheim et al. (2009a), we concluded that advice that tries to "protect sleep" by supplementing or avoiding nighttime breastfeeding is counter-productive and wrong. Unfortunately, it's the first strategy people suggest, but it's not consistent with the evidence. This is what Doan et al. (2007) said regarding their findings:

> Using supplemental as a coping strategy for minimizing sleep loss can actually be detrimental because of its impact on prolactin hormone production and secretion. . . . Maintenance of breast-feeding as well as deep restorative sleep stages may be greatly compromised for new mothers who cope with infant feedings by supplementing in an effort to get more sleep time. (p. 201)

EMERGENCY STRATEGIES FOR WHEN YOU MUST GET SOME SLEEP

At this point, you may want to continue breastfeeding but are so fatigued that you are not sure if you can. Most new mothers have been where you are. Tired is normal for this stage of your life, but "more tired" is not. Here are some strategies that might help (Goyal et al., 2007, 2009). Consider these exhaustion hacks to be emergency strategies. After a day or two, you will probably feel better and can decide whether you need to continue with them.

Four-Hour Stretch of Sleep

Our first goal is to get you 4 hours of uninterrupted sleep. This is a safe amount for your breasts and can make a huge difference in how you feel. Be sure to empty your breasts thoroughly before you go to bed. I recommend that your support person be awake, so they hear the baby before you do. If you don't know that someone is responding to the baby, you might not be able to relax enough to get to sleep. Since you need an awake support person, you may think about going to bed early (like 8 p.m.). That way, your support person can still get some sleep too, especially if they need to go to work the next day. Be sure to have some pumped milk available so your support person can feed your baby during your sleep stretch.

After 4 hours, if your baby is near you, you can handle other feedings. If you have the option to sleep in a bit in the morning, it's a good time to do so too.

Daytime Naps

Goyal et al. (2007) also found that new mothers who are depressed napped fewer than 60 minutes per day, so napping is another important strategy to help you cope with early postpartum. That might seem like a pipe dream. Even if it seems impossible, though, do what you can to move toward this goal. Enlist your support people for help. Remember that you have recently given birth and you may have had major surgery. Your body needs time to recover. Even if you haven't given birth, I've known many adoptive mothers who are exhausted postpartum. It's the nature of life with a new baby.

Napping means getting some sleep during the day, which may mean less time for other things, like housework, preparing meals, or laundry. You may need someone to watch older children. This is another time when support is essential. You can do this with your baby, or you can feed your baby, make sure they are being cared for, and just take a brief break.

CONCLUSION

In the fog of early motherhood, you may think that you will be tired for the rest of your days. That's your right brain talking, and what it's telling you is not true. I want to give your left brain something to hang on to: 40 days and 40 nights. At the end of this time, your baby goes through a huge shift in their brain development. That's a wondrous thing, and it will make it easier for you. While babies continue to defy routines, there will be some regularity to your days. The end is in sight. Accepting offers of help doesn't mean you're "weak"; it means you're sensible. I promise, life with your new baby does get easier.

CHAPTER 10

BEDSHARING AND INFANT SLEEP LOCATION

Nighttime feedings are one of the major challenges of life with a new baby. Many families decide to bring their babies to bed with them (Blair et al., 2020; McKenna, 2020). Unfortunately, they receive little guidance on how to do it safely, and some babies have died as a result. In this chapter, I describe what we know about bedsharing, when it's safe to do so, and when you need to avoid it. Where your baby sleeps has mental health implications as well, as this mother describes:

> I think that if I had done safe bedsharing from day one, my mental health wouldn't have suffered as much with being sleep deprived and trying to put a baby in a bloody cot when he hated it!

WHERE YOUR BABY SLEEPS THE FIRST 6 MONTHS

According to the American Academy of Pediatrics (2016), your baby should sleep in your room for the first 6 months, which cuts the risk of sudden infant death syndrome (SIDS) by half. Whether your baby should sleep in your bed is quite a bit more controversial. Many hospitals and public health problems in the United States (including the governmental program WIC) prohibit their employees from discussing bedsharing or cosleeping at all. The only thing they are allowed to say is "don't do it." One hospital wanted me to present on sleep and called to make sure I would be "on message." I told them I wouldn't be so suggested that they pick another topic. I did end up speaking there but did not talk about sleep. They only wanted to hear one thing. The party line is "all bedsharing is bad," which is extremely unfortunate. When providers can't talk to parents about where their babies sleep, parents unknowingly do dangerous things. In this chapter, I'll walk you through the pros and cons of bedsharing. If you decide to do it, I want it to be safe, and some parents need to avoid it completely.

THE AMERICAN ACADEMY OF PEDIATRICS' SAFE-SLEEP POLICIES

The American Academy of Pediatrics (AAP) is strongly anti-bedsharing, and have been for a long time, but their policy has evolved over the years. They will likely never support mother–infant bedsharing, but they at least now acknowledge that it happens and have offered advice to make sure that it is safe.

Here's how it started: the 2005 AAP statement (AAP Task Force on Sudden Infant Death Syndrome, 2005) was adamant about never bedsharing, ever; the baby should be in the parents' room but not in their bed. Unfortunately, the "never, ever" advice had serious consequences, like parents doing frightening things because they didn't know better. In public health speak, this is an unintended consequence. The "never, ever" advice has also resulted in some bizarre public health campaigns aimed at parents. One example was from Milwaukee and featured pictures of babies sleeping on their stomachs next to large butcher knives, saying this was "as dangerous as sleeping with your baby." In the poster, they were older babies, not infants. That's relevant because it's newborns who are most at risk. The babies on the poster were on their stomachs (not safe), with fluffy comforters (also not safe), next to gigantic knives? Who would do that?

When I was editor of *Clinical Lactation*, I wrote an editorial about that called "Don't Sleep With Big Knives" (Kendall-Tackett, 2012). We might have just laughed this off, but it failed to stop babies from dying. Within 2 months, the city of Milwaukee had two more "cosleeping" deaths. (In many parts of the Western world, any apparent case of SIDS or infant death that takes place outside of a crib is called a "cosleeping death." It's been one of the things that has plagued researchers trying to evaluate risk because some places are far more dangerous than others.) Regarding the infant deaths in Milwaukee, both babies were in highly unsafe sleeping environments (sleeping alone in an adult bed or sleeping alone with other children in two crib mattresses on the floor). There was nothing in the public health campaign that let parents know that this wasn't safe. A campaign listing safe and unsafe behaviors would have been less flashy but likely far more effective.

I became interested in studying mother–infant sleep when I started hearing from mothers and fathers that they were taking turns sleeping on the couch or recliner with their newborns to avoid bedsharing. It was hard for me not to gasp when I heard it. Sleeping on a couch or chair with a baby is much more dangerous than sleeping in a bed. I told our state director of maternal–infant health what I was hearing, and she didn't think it was really a problem. I knew we needed evidence, and that's when we launched the Survey of Mothers' Sleep and Fatigue.

Our study included 6,410 new mothers (Kendall-Tackett et al., 2010). We found that 44% of mothers admitted to falling asleep on a chair or sofa while breastfeeding at night (and those are just the mothers who admitted it). These mothers were trying to avoid bedsharing to be "safe," but falling asleep with their babies on a couch or sofa is much more dangerous (in Tappin et al.'s, 2005, study, it increased the risk of SIDS by 67 times). In our study, mothers with higher incomes and education levels were the most likely to do this.

This is a perfect example of an unintended consequence. Bad policy turned this low-risk group into a high-risk group, and mothers were engaging in a dangerous behavior to avoid bedsharing. They thought they were doing the right thing and because no one was allowed to talk to them about it, no one could tell them that it wasn't safe.

By 2011, the AAP statement was more nuanced (AAP Task Force on Sudden Infant Death Syndrome, 2011a). They acknowledged that no one should be sleeping with a baby on a sofa or chair: "Because of the extremely high risk of SIDS and suffocation on couches and armchairs, infants should not be fed on a couch or armchair when there is a high risk that the parent might fall asleep" (p. 1033).

The AAP also recommended supporting breastfeeding and avoiding the couch: "Therefore, if the infant is brought into bed for feeding, comforting, and bonding, the infant should be returned to the crib when the parent is ready for sleep" (AAP Task Force on Sudden Infant Death Syndrome, 2011b).

It was now okay to feed in bed, but they didn't account for mothers' falling asleep while nursing. By 2016, they changed their statement again (AAP, 2016). The AAP still doesn't support bedsharing, but they at least acknowledge that a mother may fall asleep while nursing. AAP stressed the importance of making sure the sleep space is safe for your baby if you happen to fall asleep. Yes!

WHAT PARENTS ARE ACTUALLY DOING

Although providers tell parents not to bedshare, most do but keep that information to themselves. A study of 1,867 women in Oregon, based on PRAMS data (Pregnancy Risk Assessment Monitory System), found that 77% of parents bedshare for at least part of the night (Lahr et al., 2007). Only 15% of White people said that they bedshare, which seems unlikely, given that they are driven by the same biological imperatives as other ethnic groups. I suspected that the data depended on how one asked the question. Our sample of 6,410 new mothers included 91% White mothers. When we asked, "Where does your baby *end* the night?" A full 60% indicated that their babies ended the night in their beds, and this was true across the entire first year (Kendall-Tackett et al., 2010). That's 4 times the number of White mothers who admitted to bedsharing in the PRAMS study (Lahr et al., 2005).

Why Parents Bedshare

When we asked why parents decided to bedshare, 60% of bedsharers reported that it was the "right thing to do," but 70% said it was the "only thing that worked." Their decisions were both pragmatic than ideologic, but respondents cited both reasons. Not surprisingly, 70% of bedsharers did not tell their health care providers (Kendall-Tackett et al., 2010).

Who Else Is in the Bed?

I also asked who else was in the bed. Bedsharers were significantly more likely to also have their partners in the bed with them (52%) than those with the baby in the room (11%) and those with babies in a separate room (29%). More worrisome was that 82% of bedsharers had other children in the bed, and 51% had their pets in the bed. Other children can work if you have a big bed, and your baby is not sleeping next to them. And as much as I love animals, I'm not sure having them in bed with an infant is ever a good idea.

BEDSHARING SUSTAINS BREASTFEEDING

For many years, SIDS and breastfeeding advocates faced off against each other. SIDS researchers claimed that breastfeeding advocates did not care about infant safety, then they discovered that breastfeeding reduced the risk of SIDS by 50% (Blair et al., 2020; Vennemann et al., 2009). What sustains breastfeeding? You got it! Bedsharing, as these mothers describe:

> Flat out discouraging bedsharing without discussing ways to do it safely undermines breastfeeding success.

> "Safe-sleep practices" of putting baby in bassinets (which I ended up co-sleeping the whole time) definitely would've made it more difficult to breastfeed.

The Academy of Breastfeeding Medicine, in its new protocol of bedsharing and breastfeeding, is even more forthright. In its opening sentence, the authors state that "bedsharing promotes breastfeeding initiation, duration, and exclusivity" (Blair et al., 2020, p. 5). Previous studies have found that to be true.

British sleep researcher Dr. Helen Ball (2007) conducted a 1-year longitudinal study of 97 mother–infant breastfeeding pairs. She found that when families bedshared, they were twice as likely to continue breastfeeding. Seventy percent of infants were bedsharing in the first month. By 6 months, 44% were still bedsharing. The same result was found in the much larger Avon Longitudinal Study of Parents and Children (ALSPAC) study from the United Kingdom ($N = 14,062$). Dr. Peter Blair and colleagues (2010) found that any type of bedsharing increased rates of breastfeeding at 12 months. They noted the following: "Advice on whether bedsharing should be discouraged needs to take into account the important relationship with breastfeeding" (p. e1119).

Dr. James McKenna, a seminal figure in mother–infant sleep, did a qualitative study of 200 mothers (McKenna & Volpe, 2007). Mothers reported that bedsharing was a "natural result" of frequent nighttime feeding. Bedsharing happened even when families planned to have their infant sleep in a crib. The ease of nighttime breastfeeding, and the emotional security of bedsharing, made it the most practical arrangement.

WHEN IS IT DANGEROUS TO BEDSHARE?

The Academy of Breastfeeding Medicine updated its protocol on bedsharing and breastfeeding. This protocol uses a risk-minimization approach, emphasizing the importance of discussing bedsharing and safe sleep with parents. The academy's approach is that breastfeeding mothers are not advised against bedsharing as long as no hazardous circumstances exist.

To understand safe sleep, it's instructive to look at studies on SIDS and sudden unexpected infant death. SIDS researchers often use case-controlled studies, where researchers assemble data on a group of infants who died, compare them with living infants who have similar demographics, and try to determine the differences. SIDS research is difficult because data are often missing. Further, sometimes researchers include deaths that happened on sofas as part of the "bedsharing" deaths, which inflates the findings.

Tappin et al. (2005) compared 123 babies who died of SIDS to 263 living infants in Scotland. Of the 123 babies, only 40 were found in their parents' beds (note that the number of deaths in cribs is substantially higher), and only 16 of those 40 were breastfeeding. In this study, all of the babies who died were less than 11 weeks old. They examined other risk factors and calculated the increased risk of SIDS for each. The risk of SIDS increased

- 12 times for babies who sleep in separate rooms with parents who smoke,
- 29 times for infants sleeping between parents,
- *67 times for sleeping on a couch or chair*, and
- 10 times for babies under 11 weeks.

Notably, they found that *bedsharing did not increase risk of death if babies were older than 11 weeks.*

Blair and Ball (2004) examined data over 3 years, with a total of 470,000 births in five regions in the United Kingdom. Of those, there were 325 cases of SIDS compared with 1,300 controls. Babies were more at risk if they weighed less than 2,500 grams (5 lb) at birth and were born before 37 weeks' gestation. Other problems were side or prone (face down) sleep positions or parents who smoked. *Bedsharing did not increase risk with nonsmoking parents and full-term babies who weighed more than 2,500 grams.*

Vennemann and colleagues (2012) pooled studies together and did a meta-analysis, which formed the basis of the AAP 2011 statement. They compared 2,404 babies who died of SIDS with 6,495 living infants (control group) and found that 29% of the SIDS group bedshared compared with 13% in the control group. They concluded that bedsharing increased the risk of SIDS by 2.89 times. However, they noted that there was "some heterogeneity in the analysis." This means that some of these data included couch or recliner sleeping, which artificially inflates the findings. These studies guide us about what not to do, but many of these findings do not separate out by feeding method. That's a problem because breastfeeding decreases SIDS risk but formula-feeding increases it.

SAFE BEDSHARING

Bedsharing can be safe within some specific parameters (Blair et al., 2020). Infant safety is the most important thing. The following sections describe what must be present for bedsharing to be safe.

The Baby Is Breastfeeding

The ABM protocol notes that mothers who have "never initiated breastfeeding" should avoid bedsharing. Stated another way, it's not safe to bedshare if you are not breastfeeding because breastfeeding changes the way you sleep. Drs. James McKenna, Helen Ball, and others (Blair et al., 2020) have documented that formula-feeding mothers sleep differently with their babies than those who are breastfeeding. The breastfeeding mother tends to sleep face-to-face with their babies, and they make a nest with their arms and curl their legs around. The fact that you see this pattern all over the world suggests biology at play.

An intensive care unit (ICU) nurse once told me that in ICUs, they blow carbon dioxide on patients' faces to stimulate breathing. A mother in this sleep position naturally does the same thing for her baby by exhaling near her baby's face. Babies are more likely to be on their backs when they sleep with their mothers but are on their sides when they nurse. This keeps them from being in one position for too long.

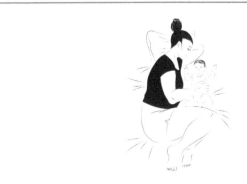

The C-position is one that breastfeeding mothers adopt all over the world when sleeping with their babies (Blair et al., 2020). Their bodies form a nest for the baby, keeping them safe. Also, the mother's body blocks anyone else who is in the bed from sleeping near the infant.

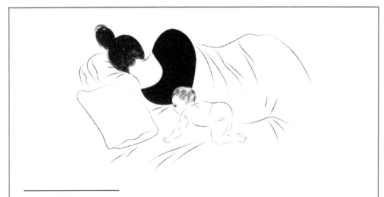

Dr. Ball's (2006) study demonstrated that women who are not breastfeeding but are sleeping with their babies do not form the nest for their babies and may even turn away while sleeping.

Whether exclusive breastfeeding is necessary for safe bedsharing is up for debate and depends on who you ask. Exclusive breastfeeding would be the safest, but a bottle or two of supplementation may not influence the behavior that keeps babies safe. It's a judgment call, and some mothers find it's also a great way for them to reconnect with their babies if they've been apart all day.

The Mother and Her Partner Do Not Smoke

Smoking increases the risk of SIDS by up to 10 times (Tappin et al., 2005), so bedsharing is not safe if you smoke, even if you're breastfeeding (Blair et al., 2020). Researchers don't know exactly why smoking and bedsharing are a dangerous combination, but they are. Is it the nicotine in the milk? Is it the smoke residue on the mother's or her partner's hair and skin? Is it all of the above? We're not sure, but the elevated risk is undeniable.

I learned from public health officials in New Zealand that the Indigenous Maori tribe bedshare and smoke and have a high SIDS rate. Public health officials encouraged them to weave traditional baskets and put the basket in their beds. It was a separate sleeping space, and the baby was close by. That simple intervention cut the SIDS risk in half. To have your baby near, you could consider a similar solution.

The Mother's Body Is Between Her Baby and Anyone Else in the Bed

This is a good rule of thumb, especially if you have other children in your bed. You don't want anyone else in between you and your baby. If you move your baby to your other side, make sure that they are not sleeping next to another child because that is dangerous.

Keep Your Baby Away From Anything That Might Smother Them

Don't have fluffy pillows, comforters, or blankets around where your baby sleeps (Blair et al., 2020). Put them in a one-piece sleeper so that they don't need a blanket. If you have a pillowtop or memory-foam mattress (be careful with anything that leaves an indent when you push your hand into it), make sure that the surface is firm. If you have a soft or memory-foam mattress, slide a yoga mat under your sheet, it will give you a firm surface that is safe for your baby.

Make Sure Your Bed Is Not Up Against a Surface Such as a Wall or Dresser

You don't want your baby to get stuck or wedged because they can suffocate. That is also why it is so dangerous for you to nurse on a recliner or couch. Some parents use a mesh rail that they slide on their bed if they are worried that their baby may fall out. If you use a rail, make sure it is a tight fit so that your baby cannot slide between the bed and the rail.

Don't Put Your Baby Prone (Face Down)

When babies sleep on separate surfaces, people often want to put them prone (face down) so that they don't startle themselves awake. (When you watch your baby, you can definitely see that.) On the basis of what we know now, back sleeping seems to be safest. (Some practitioners worry about babies' development if they are always on their backs. You can minimize potential negative effects by using a sling during the day and having your baby in a variety of positions during the day. That way, they are not always on their back.)

Make Sure That Your Baby Is Warm but Not Too Warm

Overheating can increase the risk of SIDS. Dressing your baby in a sleeper ensures that your baby is warm without a blanket.

Never Bedshare if You Have Taken Something That Can Impair Your Ability to Respond

This is critical. Safe bedsharing depends on your being able to respond to your baby at night. If you take anything that makes you sleepy, including alcohol, cannabis, recreational drugs, or prescription medications, your baby needs to sleep in a separate space (Blair et al., 2020; Blair et al., 2006; McKenna, 2020). Period.

I remember hearing about a particularly tragic case. A mother had had a cesarean and was given morphine, which would be appropriate to control her pain. Someone at the hospital tucked the baby in with the mother and didn't stay there to watch her. The baby died.

Another time, I was lecturing in the Midwest, and they had a particularly vehement anti-bedsharing campaign. I sat next to the architect of that plan during dinner. They had had seven infant deaths in 6 months. I learned that six of the seven deaths involved substance use and none of the mothers were breastfeeding. These cases were completely different from a nonimpaired, nonsmoking, breastfeeding mother. I'm happy to say that she told me that she decided to rethink her policy.

IF YOU CAN'T BEDSHARE

If you can't have your baby in bed, you may still want to keep them close to handle night feedings. One mom recently moved to our community and was staying in a residence hotel until their house was ready. Her baby was in their room but on the other side and was having to get out of bed and walk across the room to get him, which was wearing her out. Just moving the bassinet closer helped. She didn't have to completely wake up to respond to her baby.

It will be easier if your baby is on the same level as you, especially if you've had a cesarean section or difficult vaginal birth. Having your baby at your same height puts less pressure on these tender spots and will be safer for you to lift. Here are some other suggestions that mothers have found to be helpful.

Options for Non-Bedsharing

Your Pack 'n Play is next to your bed, the crib is next to your bed, or use a cosleeper. Make sure that there are no gaps between the

155

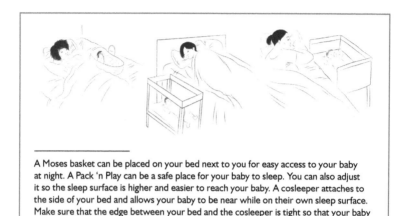

A Moses basket can be placed on your bed next to you for easy access to your baby at night. A Pack 'n Play can be a safe place for your baby to sleep. You can also adjust it so the sleep surface is higher and easier to reach your baby. A cosleeper attaches to the side of your bed and allows your baby to be near while on their own sleep surface. Make sure that the edge between your bed and the cosleeper is tight so that your baby cannot fall in between.

cosleeper and the side of your bed. A final option is a basket you place in your bed, which also gives your baby a separate sleep surface but is handy for you.

IN SOME CASES, BEDSHARING MAY BE BAD FOR YOUR MENTAL HEALTH

You won't see this in another breastfeeding book, but you need to know about our findings on bedsharing and mothers' mental health (Kendall-Tackett et al., 2018). Bedsharing may not be a good idea for mixed-feeding mothers. In our sample, mothers self-identified as exclusive breastfeeding, mixed-feeding, or formula-feeding. As with our earlier findings, there was no significant difference between mixed- and formula-feeding mothers. Practically speaking, how many bottles does it take to make bedsharing risky? One a day? Two? Three or more? We don't actually know. This may come down to your judgment. If you are mixed-feeding and bedsharing, you are breastfeeding enough to make it safe for your baby (Blair et al., 2020), but bedsharing could be having a negative effect on you. See if these findings are relevant for you.

Bedsharing and Sleep Time

Exclusively breastfeeding (EBF)–bedsharing mothers got the most sleep, but bedsharing/non-EBF mother got the *least* amount (6.72 hours for EBF vs. 6.18 hours for non-EBF). If you're not EBF, bedsharing may not help you at night (Kendall-Tackett, Cong, & Hale, 2018).

Mothers' Anxiety

Mothers were asked how often they were anxious or afraid. Anxiety was highest for the bedsharing–non-EBF mothers (1.2 for non-EBF vs. 0.94 for EBF). Exclusively breastfeeding mothers had lower anxiety, regardless of the baby's sleep location (Kendall-Tackett, Cong, & Hale, 2018).

Mothers' Anger and Irritability

Non-EBF–bedsharing mothers had the highest rates of anger and irritability (1.62 for non-EBF vs. 1.5 for EBF). The second highest was the non-EBF–non-bedsharing mothers (1.54). There findings are consistent with the effect of oxytocin, which decreases anger but also helps settle the baby more easily. The lowest rates of anger were for the EBF mothers, regardless of sleep location (but note that they still had some anger and irritably. Oxytocin doesn't fix everything).

157

Mothers' Depressive Symptoms

The final variable was mothers' depressive symptoms, which were lowest for EBF mothers regardless of sleep location (0.84 to 0.87 for EBF mothers). Non-EBF–non-bedsharing had the highest depressive symptoms (1.18; Kendall-Tackett, Cong, & Hale, 2018). I thought these findings were interesting because many mental health providers actually recommend this: not bedsharing and not exclusively breast-feeding. In light of our findings, that advice is not sound.

Is Bedsharing Affecting Your Mental Health?

If you're not exclusively breastfeeding, you might consider avoiding bedsharing. In practical terms, I suspect this is a gray area. Is bed-sharing working for you? Are you getting a good night's sleep? Bedsharing can reconnect you with your baby, especially if you are separated during the day, but if you are mostly formula-feeding, you might find that it works better for you to have your baby sleep near you rather than with you. However, if you are doing a lot of your breastfeeding at night, bedsharing might be just the thing.

SOME THOUGHTS ABOUT SLEEP TRAINING

When parents want to know more about infant nighttime needs, people will inevitably mention sleep training. If there is a concern about your mental health, a lot of people will recommend it. Some providers insist that you need to protect your mental health. I was recently on a panel where a fellow psychologist described how she uses cognitive therapy to help mothers not attend to their infants' nighttime needs. With all these people recommending it, we just have to ask: Does this prevent depression? The short answer is "no."

Let's look at a couple of key studies. The first was a pro–sleep-training article that made headlines worldwide (Price et al., 2012). Researchers taught mothers how to sleep train their 8- to 9-month-olds, and then followed up with the parents when their babies were 5. The researchers found no apparent harm in sleep training and thought it could be "safely recommended to parents." They also found "no apparent benefit," so why do it? It's a lot of work. More to the point, sleep training did not result in lower rates of postpartum depression.

The second article was a review of 43 studies and was sponsored by the UK National Institute of Health Research (Douglas & Hill, 2013). The researchers found that infant sleep interventions in the first 6 months did not reduce infant crying, prevent sleep and behavioral problems in later childhood, or prevent postpartum depression. Instead, they found unintended consequences of sleep training, including increased problem crying, premature cessation of breastfeeding, worsened maternal anxiety, and increased risk for SIDS. They concluded that an evidence-based approach to sleep problems avoids both extinction and graduated extinction, two forms of sleep training.

Dr. Wendy Middlemiss and colleagues (2011, 2017) studied mothers and babies who enrolled in a 5-day residential program in New Zealand, where they sleep-trained babies for parents. At the beginning of the study, mothers and babies were hormonally in sync (cortisol levels for both mothers and babies were high). By Day 3, they were no longer in sync. Babies were stressed, but mothers were not. Dr. Middlemiss considered this lack of synchrony one of her most ominous findings; mothers were out of touch with their babies. By Day 5, babies were no longer crying, so people might call that a success. However, the babies had high cortisol levels, a sign of stress, but were no longer asking for help. To me, there is something tragic about these stressed, mute babies (see next section).

159

MY CONCERNS ABOUT SLEEP TRAINING

I've always approached sleep training from the perspective of a stress and trauma researcher. From my work, I know that chronically high stress is not good for adult brains. The effects are even more profound for infants, whose nervous systems are still developing. This makes them even more vulnerable. Sleep training raises some serious concerns for me.

Secure Attachment

Responsive care is the bedrock of forming a secure attachment and that does not switch off at night. Ignoring a baby's cries could affect attachment (Middlemiss & Kendall-Tackett, 2014; Narvaez, 2013). A lot would depend on the type of training and how long it went on, but chronically ignoring a baby's cries will have an impact. This is true even beyond the newborn period. For example, babies who have been sleeping through the night often start waking again around 9 months. This sudden night-waking coincides with something developmentalists call baby's developing "object permanence." They can still imagine that something exists even when they can't see it. They now know you exist even when they can't see you. At this age, if they wake up and you are not there, to their baby brain, they've been abandoned and they cry out for you. They are expressing a real need. Unfortunately, this is a key age when parents turn to sleep training.

How did parents handle older babies' nighttime needs in our study? We saw an interesting pattern. At about 6 months, many babies were moved into their own rooms. However, 60% of parents said that their babies *ended* the night in their beds and that was true throughout the first year. Babies started out alone, but when they woke, they were brought into bed rather than left to cry alone (Kendall-Tackett et al., 2010). Parents probably never discussed this with anyone. They just did it.

Brain Development

In his classic paper "Why Stress Is Bad for Your Brain," stress researcher Dr. Robert Sapolsky (1996) outlined why the stress hormone cortisol hurts the brain. Most of the studies were on adults who were harmed by chronically high cortisol levels, such as with someone who has chronic depression or posttraumatic stress disorder. Cortisol actually shrinks cells in a part of the brain called the hippocampus, the seat of learning and memory. This happens even when they put hippocampal cells in a Petri dish and drip cortisol on them; the cells shrink. As I described earlier, babies' developing brains are far more vulnerable. Shonkoff et al. (2009) went further by describing how early toxic stress sets people up for a lifetime of health problems and that avoiding early toxic stress means better health throughout the lifespan. Sleep training increases cortisol (Buss et al., 2012; Narvaez, 2013). For me, that's a strong argument against sleep training; I'm in favor of avoiding all practices that elevate cortisol in prolonged way.

Milk Production

In the early weeks, limiting nighttime feeds can lower your milk production. In addition, babies need to eat at night or their weight may falter. Moreover, if you cut nighttime feedings, you won't empty your breasts as often as you need. That will be less true as your baby matures, but it is a consideration while you are establishing your supply.

CONCLUSION

Bedsharing has been practiced throughout human history—even historically in the United States. It can be a practical solution to feeding your baby at night and coping with the early weeks of motherhood. Many families also enjoy the closeness of having their babies near them at night (McKenna & Volpe, 2007).

As lovely as bedsharing can be, it's also important to be safe, and in some cases, you may need to avoid it for the sake of both safety and your mental health. I would still encourage you to have your baby near you and, per the AAP guidelines, strongly encourage you to have your baby in your room for the first 6 months because this cuts the risk of SIDS in half (AAP, 2016). With your baby nearby, you can respond to their needs and get some sleep, which is always a good thing and the easiest way to get through your first few weeks as a new parent.

V

FINDING BREASTFEEDING SUPPORT

INTRODUCTION: FINDING BREASTFEEDING SUPPORT

Finding support is critical to your success with breastfeeding, but as with any human relationship, we must wade through the messy bits to get there. The construct of social support has two main components: the supportive action and your *perception* of the action. In other words, did it feel like support to you? Here's an example: cleaning someone's home. Generally speaking, that's a kind act. Doing it for a new mother allows her to rest and focus on her baby. However, what if the mother feels judged, or what if there is a silent, or even spoken, question of "why aren't you doing this yourself?" or "I didn't have help after I had a baby. You're lucky." In this context, "help" doesn't feel good and can even make a mother feel "lazy."

TYPES OF BREASTFEEDING SUPPORT

The same can be true for breastfeeding support. It can take many forms. Information at just the right time. Reassurance that things are going well or empathy when they are not. Practical help such as picking up groceries, doing the dishes, or watching your baby so you can take a shower.

Davidson and Ollerton (2020) reviewed eight articles on partner support for breastfeeding. Their findings are relevant to all types of support because they get at the fundamental structure: supportive action and perception of the action. When partners offered help and encouragement, breastfeeding initiation increased, but women sometimes had negative views of "help and encouragement."

Responsiveness was the most effective kind of support and included being sensitive to women's needs, respecting their decisions, and promoting self-efficacy. If partners took mothers' needs seriously and mothers and partners acted together as a team, breastfeeding initiation, exclusivity, and duration increased. When partners offered knowledge, help, and encouragement without responsiveness, breastfeeding duration decreased. With responsiveness, women felt understood, validated, and cared for. Without responsiveness, practical support meant that they are not self-sufficient, and encouragement felt like coercion to breastfeed or meet impossible breastfeeding goals.

Another recent study examined women's networks of breastfeeding support (Emmott et al., 2020). This study was conducted in the United Kingdom, which has one of the lowest breastfeeding rates in Europe, and included 432 mothers. The researchers identified three types of support networks. The first was *Extensive Support*, where mothers had support from partners, their mother, friends, and health professionals. In this group, only the mother fed the baby. The second group was *Family Support*, where the mothers had support from their partners and mothers but had little support from health care providers. Partners and grandmothers also fed the baby. The final group was called *Low Support*, where the support was primarily from partners. Mothers fed their babies.

At 2 months postpartum, 94% of the mothers in the *Extensive Support* group were still breastfeeding, demonstrating the old maxim "It takes a village." The next highest was the supposed *Low Support* group, with 48% still breastfeeding. The *Family Support* group had, by far, the lowest rates of breastfeeding (only 13%), and it demonstrates what happens when others step in to feed the baby in the first 2 months: breastfeeding rates plummet. Unfortunately, many mental health providers recommend this approach, and it's usually a disaster for breastfeeding.

HOW FAMILY AND FRIENDS CAN HELP EFFECTIVELY

In *Breastfeeding Uncovered*, Dr. Amy Brown (2016) described how friends, family, and others can undermine breastfeeding in some subtle ways.

- Your mother tells you that she fed you every four hours and you are fine.
- Your mother-in-law insists on holding the baby a little longer and not giving him back.
- Your partner wants to bond with the baby and sees feeding as the only way.
- You buy a book that tells you when babies should be fed (and it's not now).
- You feel so exhausted your health visitor suggests that your partner does a feed.
- A mom at the baby clinic asks if your milk is enough because he's feeding so much.
- Your friends without children want you to go out for a break from the baby. (pp. 70–72)

In contrast, she suggested some things they can that will support breastfeeding. Amy continues: "What if we lived in a society in which a mum's job is to feed her baby when it needs feeding, and the rest of the world supports her doing that? What if?"

- Rather than wanting to feed the baby himself, dad cooks a lovely meal for everyone (which kind of feeds the baby anyway)?
- Your mother passes the baby back to you and makes you a cup of tea (with biscuits)?

167

- Society just gets on with their coffee, cake, and gossip and doesn't even notice a mother breastfeeding her baby, as it's so normal?
- Friends come round to the house, tidy up a bit and hold the sleeping baby for you while you have a moment hands-free?
- Someone writes a parenting manual that simply says, "feed and cuddle your baby whenever you both want. The end" (short book maybe, but priceless). (pp. 71–73)

Social support is in the eye of the beholder; your perception is the most important thing. If it doesn't feel like support, it isn't. And if you need it, I'm giving you permission to limit your exposure to unsupportive people. Your comfort and happiness are the most important elements to make this work. I hope these chapters will steer you through the challenges and help you assemble the support network you need.

CHAPTER 11

FAMILY AND COMMUNITY SUPPORT

Support makes everything better. The goal of this chapter is to help you find support from your friends, family, and community. I want you to have a strong network that can get you through the early days.

> I strongly believe it's all about your support system those first few weeks are hard. . . . The more access to support and resources, the better. (Mother in our survey)

RELATIVES AND FRIENDS

Friends and family can improve our lives and help us live longer. We're meant to go through life in a caravan. And as with any type of human experience, your nearest and dearest can support or derail your breastfeeding efforts. They may want to help but don't know how, or they might feel left out or threatened because you are doing something different. The next three chapters include some ideas on how to make social support work. These chapters can also help you ask for the type of support that you need.

Partners

For many new mothers, partners are the first place they turn, and they are the persons most associated with breastfeeding success. Without partner support, breastfeeding often ends prematurely. They are critical to this enterprise, yet we often exclude partners or tell them to change diapers, which diminishes their important role. Lactation providers need to support partners as well as mothers. Ideally, mothers and their partners will work as a team, as Davidson and Ollerton (2020) described:

> When the woman and her partner work together as a "breast-feeding team," effective supportive behaviours are more likely to occur and result in improved autonomy and self-efficacy of mothers and their partners as well as in improved breast-feeding outcomes. *Teamwork may, therefore, be the core aspect of responsive breastfeeding support, reflecting a key element of effective social support evident within the sociological literature.* (p. e22, emphasis added)

In a review of 27 studies on fathers' support for breastfeeding, Ngoenthong and colleagues (2020) found that fathers believed breastfeeding was necessary for infants, but they felt left out and useless. Fathers were more likely to feel negatively about breastfeeding when they felt helpless, anxious, guilty, or unable to assist their partners in overcoming difficulties. They felt that they had few opportunities to bond with their breastfeeding baby and were invisible in their antenatal classes. The authors concluded that fathers need support and information so that they can support their partners. Without that, mothers are more likely to stop breastfeeding early. This article was written about fathers, but most of these feelings are relevant to same-sex partners. In some ways, same-sex partners are even more invisible. One same-sex partner told me that she didn't even feel like a parent. It helped when she was included in breastfeeding support.

During the early weeks, the mother–baby bond becomes all-consuming. Especially as breastfeeding is being established, partners can feel like a third wheel. Fortunately, there is much that partners can do to be part of the action. Following are some suggestions. If you are a partner reading this, please know that you are critical to making breastfeeding work.

What Partners Can Do to Help

- *Take notes during visits with the lactation consultant or physician.* Mothers are in right-brain mode in the early days, and it's hard to listen to left-brain instructions. Partners can be the left-brain in the family.
- *Be an extra set of hands.* An interesting development during COVID has been lactation consulting via Zoom. When we're in person, there's always the temptation to "help" with our hands. During COVID, we couldn't do that, and it's been a surprisingly good thing. Partners can move the phone or computer for a good angle, for example, or check to ensure that the bottom lip is not tucked under, something mothers can't see. This makes breastfeeding a couples' activity, and when it works, they both can feel proud.
- *Give Mom a break so she can take a shower or get a nap.* Babies' needs are intense, so it's great if she can share the load. Partners don't need to feed their babies to hang out with and get to know them.
- *Screen visitors and calls, and protect the mother from unhelpful advice.* Unsolicited advice is a real challenge. Mothers need the confidence to meet their breastfeeding goals, and it is fragile in

the beginning. If someone makes the mother doubt her abilities, it can undermine her success. Protecting her from unhelpful advice is a real service.

- *Know when a baby is getting enough to eat.* Reassure the mother or seek help if necessary. Partners can help by knowing when the baby is getting enough to eat. That is a left-brain activity (counting daily feeds or poopy diapers). If there are signs of trouble, they can find help, make an appointment, and write down any instructions.

- *Work with the mother to interact with health care providers.* Health care providers can support or undermine breastfeeding. As I describe in the next chapter, their personal experiences may have been negative, or they have a parenting style that conflicts with yours. Their advice may be outdated or not evidence based. Partners can help mothers discern whether the advice is sound.

- *Bond with the baby in other ways than feeding.* Many new parents can't wait to feed their babies, and I understand why. It's a special time. The good news is that you don't need to feed the baby to bond. I suggest that partners wait at least 4 weeks until the mother's milk production is firmly established before feeding the baby. This advice also applies to partners who want to conurse.

    Instead of feeding, partners might try skin-to-skin contact or babywearing, bathing the baby, doing infant massage, or going outside for a walk. Your baby knows your partner's voice. Doula and childbirth educator Penny Simkin tells how she teaches partners of expectant mothers to sing to their babies in utero. Once the baby is born, babies turn and react to their partner's voice. Talk to your baby, make eye contact, and engage with them. All of these activities will help establish your unique relationship with your baby.

Your Mother

Whether good or bad, your relationship with your mother will likely amplify now that you have your own baby. Some women find that their mothers are important to their breastfeeding success. In our survey, 7% said their mother was the most helpful person to support breastfeeding. If your mother is no longer in your life, you may especially miss her during this time.

> The people who were the most help were my mother and sister. They both breastfed and I called them constantly until my nipples were used to breastfeeding. Having a support group is key to having a good experience I believe.

> I was 18 when I had my baby. The doctor/hospital was terrible about teaching me how to do anything. Everything I learned . . . was taught to me by my mom.

These mothers also found that their mothers were key in their breastfeeding success. They provided practical, informational, and emotional support.

> My baby was 6 weeks early. The nurse casually suggested I start pumping since she was in the ICU, but I was so disoriented from the last-minute surgery and pain drugs that I did not understand. The only reason I was able to breastfeed was that my mother intervened and made sure I was pumping. She found lactation consultants and stayed on top of it checking in every few hours. If she had not done that, my milk would have dried up. Breastfeeding was crucial to helping my baby and I bond after 10 days in the ICU and probably is the reason she started to grow so well.

> My mother is an IBCLC [International Board Certified Lactation Consultant], and she helped me daily once I was discharged.

I don't know if I would have been as successful if I didn't have the daily, hands-on encouragement and support.

In contrast, 16% of the mothers in our survey reported that their mother was the *least helpful person* when learning to breast-feed. During the early days of breastfeeding, you may run into issues with your mother. Why might this occur?

- *Your parenting choices differ.* If you are breastfeeding and she did not, she may feel defensive and say something like, "I didn't breastfeed you, and you are fine." Perhaps she wanted to breast-feed but couldn't because of lack of support, bad advice, or a medical condition that precluded it. She may be grieving her lack of ability to meet her own breastfeeding goals. She may have also made different parenting decisions regarding circum-cision, cosleeping, babywearing, or answering babies' cries.

- *Sometimes mothers do not understand how breastfeeding works or may be using outdated information.* While breast-feeding doesn't change, what we know about it does. As we learn more, we have better knowledge about helping mothers. Granted, sometimes the old information works better than the new. If your mother has breastfeeding advice, you might try what she suggests because it could be just the thing. You might also share what you have learned. Ideally, you can work together to come up with a solution for whatever challenge you face.

- *Her information might not be helpful.* An example can be applying a bottle-feeding norm to a breastfeeding situation. Breastfeeding differs in every way from exclusive formula-feeding. There is no schedule for breastfeeding. It's based on responding to the baby's hunger cues rather than the clock. If you've always known formula, this will seem chaotic. Your mother may worry that your baby is not getting enough if they are on the breast "all the time."

- *Your mother may be genuinely concerned about you if you are having breastfeeding problems.* I understand her concern, but she might propose skipping breastfeeding instead. Let's assume good intent here. She is looking out for your welfare.
- *If possible, it's best to have your mother on your side.* You can share with her your breastfeeding goals and enlist your partner in these discussions. Come up with some ways that she truly can contribute.
- *If your relationship with your mother has been difficult, or if there has been abuse, neglect, or other dysfunction, postpartum may exacerbate these difficulties.* In this case, you may need to limit your contact with your mother during these early weeks. Enlist your partner and others in your support network, including a postpartum doula. It is okay for you to limit negative influences, especially in the early weeks.

Other Relatives

Members of your extended family can complicate things even further. Best-case scenario, they are there to help. Unfortunately, it might not be quite so easy. Your relationship with your mother-in-law can also be challenging. Your parenting choices may differ from hers or she may feel that you are judging her choices, or she may be a big help.

The same goes for other family members, and this often starts in the hospital when they crowd into the hospital room, which can make it difficult for you to rest and learn to breastfeed. You might not feel comfortable revealing your breasts. Another interesting lesson from COVID-19 is that visitation was severely limited. This is completely anecdotal, but many of my nurse and lactation consultant friends across the United States told me that limited visitation made it easier for the mothers to get breastfeeding off to a good start. There were, obviously, many downsides to what happened during COVID, so this observation was a surprise.

If family members are helpful to you, by all means, involve them in your day-to-day life, especially if they come bearing a casserole or are willing to throw in a load of laundry. If, however, they are making you anxious, questioning your parenting choices, offering unsolicited advice, or expecting you to wait on them, then it's okay to create some distance. Your partner, support person, or postpartum doula can help. It's better for the baby not to be exposed to a lot of people in the first few weeks anyway. Ask yourself honestly, "Is this person helpful and do I enjoy seeing them? Or do I feel criticized?" If your gut says "no," it's okay to limit the number and duration of their visits. Think of it as an investment in your and your baby's well-being.

COMMUNITY SUPPORT

According to the World Health Organization's (n.d.) "10 Steps to Successful Breastfeeding," mothers need breastfeeding support in their communities, yet this is where we are often the weakest. Volunteers have stepped into this vacuum and are essential, for without them, many mothers would have no support. However, in most communities, especially in the United States, there is no national organized system of support, and support that does exist is often a patchwork of poorly funded organizations. I've worked in this segment for much of my career, and I know the incredible dedication of these organizations. I'm not criticizing them. My issue is with many hospital administrators, insurance companies, and policymakers who say they support breastfeeding but do not provide the money to make community support happen. Things could radically change for the better if they got on board.

The U.S. WIC program (the supplemental feeding program for pregnant women, infants, and children) has sponsored a hugely successful breastfeeding peer-counselor program that has increased the breastfeeding rates for lower-income mothers. With WIC in place, we see an interesting paradox: lower-income mothers often have better support than middle-class mothers who have the means to pay for support but cannot find it. It shows what a well-organized system can do.

I would like to describe two sources of community support in this chapter: mother-to-mother support organizations and social media. I'll describe professional support in the next chapter.

Mother-to-Mother Support Organizations

Mother-to-mother support organizations provide support in many forms: helplines, support groups, parenting classes, or drop-in baby cafes. I've spoken with thousands of mothers over the years who have told me that these support organizations saved them as they navigated the early days of motherhood. I know hundreds of women my age or older who made lifelong friends in these groups.

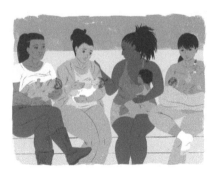

Mother-to-mother groups can offer an important source of camaraderie in addition to information and practical support.

The grandmother of these organizations is La Leche League International (LLL). Historically, La Leche League has been credited with rescuing breastfeeding when it was close to dying out in the United States and around the world. In addition to LLL, there are groups for almost everyone, so I encourage you to shop around. Depending on where you live, you usually have options.

> I was determined to breastfeed from the beginning and sought out support from LLL because my in-laws and husband encouraged me to. Without that support or LLL, things would probably have been different.

When groups go well, oxytocin flows to everyone in the room—even the helpers. These groups, however, can have a downside. Mothers can exhibit certain brinksmanship over lots of irrelevant stuff, turning everything into a competition, such as whether your baby is sleeping through the night, how much weight your baby gained, whether your baby has organic snacks. I want to shout "It's not a competition!" But it *feels* that way and can take an iron will to resist it.

In the end, these competitions are such a waste of time. You don't need to compete with other mothers—ever. You are making decisions that are right for you and your family, and that's no one else's business. It's also potentially harmful if you try to make your baby conform to someone else's. I remember one particularly awful incident. A mother with a baby about the same age as my oldest son watched me put him down for a nap at church. He happened to be tired and went right to sleep. She decided that her son needed to do that too and forced the issue, so he cried for 45 minutes straight. His kindhearted dad told me that it was "brutal." I felt sick to my stomach. It wasn't a competition, but she turned it into one, and her baby suffered for it.

If you don't like formal groups, drop-in clinics, such as Baby Cafés, can help. Many new mothers like these better than traditional support groups. You can get the information and support you need and then pop back out. See if that option is available in your community (in the United States, see https://www.babycafeusa.org, but they are worldwide).

Here's my bottom line. If you come home feeling depleted rather than uplifted or you consistently get wrong advice, steer clear. You don't need to get bogged down in an unhelpful group. A group might work well for a season, but eventually, it no longer fits. Try a few and go where you are comfortable. When they work, they tend to work well.

Social Media

In *The Virtual Breastfeeding Culture*, Lara Audelo (2013) described how mothers often use social media to get information and support about breastfeeding. In Audelo's case, her military husband was deployed when her babies were born. They moved frequently, and support was not readily available. Her online friends got her through her initial challenges, and many of these women became friends IRL (in real life).

One woman in her book was super anxious as she was wheeled into the operating room to have a cesarean. Her OB let her keep her cellphone, and she live chatted on Facebook during her surgery. A mother in our survey described the support she received from her online group.

> I did not leave the hospital feeling confident. This was my second baby to breastfeed. What helped most was a post-discharge home visit from a lactation consultant. . . . Also being part of a large Facebook group about breastfeeding mothers (I'm a physician) . . . that helped answer questions was very helpful too.

Not surprisingly, online support varies widely in terms of quality and helpfulness. Several of my younger colleagues have had negative experiences on some of those sites. I've read through a few forums myself and have been struck by the level of vitriol on some of them. Moderated forums are usually better. Breastfeeding inspires a great deal of passion, but that can turn into aggression on some sites. In addition, you have to be careful about the accuracy of the information. Industry is not silent here. Formula marketing is especially effective on social media. Remember, they make money when breastfeeding fails.

I'd suggest being cautious even when you are on a site sponsored by a company that supports breastfeeding. Although I believe most of these companies are altruistic, their goal is to sell you something. In general, I can tell you that the breastfeeding world has never been entirely comfortable with for-profit businesses that sell breastfeeding products. Many of these products are genuinely useful, but they need to sell things to survive. It doesn't mean that they're bad or are trying to trick you; it just means that their goal differs from those of a noncommercial entity. My advice is to consider the accuracy of all information, even if it is published by a breastfeeding-friendly company.

A Caution About Your Phone

Although I understand the need to stay connected, I suggest that you limit your phone time when you are with your baby. When you are hunched over your phone, you mimic the symptoms of depression. If you want to see how that looks, check out the Still-Face Mother experiments on YouTube. That was a series of studies by Dr. Edward Tronick at Children's Hospital in Boston. He was trying to mimic what happens when mothers are depressed and how that influences babies. Not surprisingly, when mothers disengage, it's stressful for babies. Being glued to your phone all day is similar to being a Still-Face Mother.

In addition, according to oxytocin researcher, Dr. Kerstin Uvnäs Moberg (personal communication, January 25, 2021), when you are engaged with your computer or your phone, you activate your stress response, which suppresses oxytocin, puts you at higher risk for depression, and can make breastfeeding more difficult. As I suggested earlier, you might consider limiting your phone time to 2 hours a day. That's enough time to be connected while still giving you time to connect with your baby in real life.

CONCLUSION

Finding support is critical to meeting your breastfeeding goals. For most new mothers, partners are the primary source of support. However, if they are not available or not helpful, finding a family member or friend to help you will make a huge difference. Many mothers find that mother-to-mother support organizations are critical to their success, especially if family and friends are not helpful. Finally, online support can also help, especially if you are isolated. The most important thing for you to do is to seek out people who empower and help you and build your network from there.

CHAPTER 12

HOSPITAL, HEALTH CARE PROVIDER, AND LACTATION CONSULTANT SUPPORT

Family members are important sources of support, but when health care providers are on board too, breastfeeding rates double (Emmott et al., 2020). This chapter focuses on support from hospitals, physicians, and lactation consultants. The ideal is a seamless system between the hospital and the community. As you will see from these mothers' stories, that happens sometimes, but the system of care is often haphazard. This isn't true of all communities. As I've traveled, I've been amazed at some of the systems different communities have put in place (the U.S. state of Kansas is a great example). That usually happens because providers have brought all the stakeholders to the table to ensure that no mother falls through the cracks. Unfortunately, that isn't the norm. Your journey may feel erratic, but support is out there. I want to help you find it.

HOSPITAL LACTATION CARE

Professional lactation support generally begins in the hospital. The system is better than it used to be but still falls short for many mothers. In the best-case scenario, all hospital staff have had lactation training, eliminating the problem of everyone telling mothers something different. In an ideal system, there is enough staff to see every mother, including nighttime and weekend coverage.

Mothers' Perceptions of Hospital Lactation Care

Mothers in our survey had a lot to say about the support that they received in the hospital. Some of the mothers reported amazing experiences:

> BEST hospital staff on the planet I'm pretty sure :) so helpful with everything, and [they] called to check up on how the breastfeeding was going a couple of times.

> My baby had latch issues so even though the hospital staff was amazing, I was still having issues feeding my baby when we left the hospital.

> I had an amazing nurse with the birth of my first that really helped me with all three of my babies.

This mother had a great experience with her hospital support group.

> We were extremely fortunate at the hospital to have a breast-feeding support group. If the [provider] hadn't taken us to it, I don't know what our breastfeeding journey would have been like. I've attended almost weekly breastfeeding support groups (now online) for the last 15 months on our feeding journey and the support is brilliant.

Although 71% of mothers in our survey said they had positive birth experiences, many were not happy with the hospital lactation support.

Lack of IBCLC [International Board Certified Lactation Consultant] coverage at hospital and pediatrician was disappointing.

We had to go to an outside lactation consultant because the ones at our hospital were terrible.

Due to COVID restrictions, I did not receive any lactation services while in the hospital or after discharge.

For my oldest son, I had an incredibly negative experience with breastfeeding. It was really hard. He didn't latch well, and I had a lactation consultant who blamed me for not knowing what to do. The second lactation consultant I saw was better, but I also felt there was a lot of pressure to breastfeed and to turn breastfeeding into this money-making scheme.

This mother described how nurses seemed more concerned with their routines than they were for her. She did not get the help she needed in the hospital.

When I asked for nurses to help me nurse, they were more interested in whether or not I had pooped (and taken laxative to help me poop). I remember so vividly asking for help as the nurse had extended her arm with laxatives in her hand, like shoving it at me. I was furious and felt completely unheard. I was seen by IBCLC in hospital, but she didn't really help me. My son had a tongue-tie that went undiagnosed for 10 days. By then, I was so damaged physically and emotionally.

Lactation Consultant Staffing

Staffing can affect the support you receive in the hospital. If there are enough lactation consultants on staff, you are likely to get good support. If the hospital does not have enough lactation staff, you may not get good support. Time is a key component of lactation support. Lactation consultants need time to sit with you and see how things are going. If the hospital has not hired enough people, the lactation consultants may run themselves ragged and need to limit how much time they can spend with you. A friend who worked at a large hospital in Boston told me that they could only spend 15 minutes with each mother, which is not nearly enough.

Lactation consultants don't like the lack of staffing either because they know what good care is and that they are not able to provide it. The result can be care like this mother described:

> I talked to the [lactation consultant] at my hospital for all of five minutes. If this wasn't my third child (I breastfed my others successfully for over a year), I would have been lost with her guidance.

Another mother described how the hospital IBCLC did not have time to wait until her baby woke up to feed:

> The IBCLC in the hospital came while my baby was sleeping and said if "I didn't work with her now, she wouldn't have time to come back at feeding time," then proceeded to rush me. I left the hospital with blistered and bruised nipples. The left is actually scarred. I had taken a hospital course and was able to use nurses to get better until I saw the lactation consultant at the peds office.

Staff know that mothers often leave before the hospital staff can determine whether breastfeeding is going well. Nurses have lots of things they need to review with you before you go. A lot of the information they share may not even register with you.

> I answered based on my first birth, in the hospital ([hospital name] a "baby friendly" hospital—ha! NOT very friendly at

the time—era of drive-thru deliveries). I had 24 hours to leave from the moment I gave birth . . . regardless of how long I'd been in labor prior. My second birth was TOTALLY different—home birth, support, and wonderful info every step of the way!

Short staffing can also influence when care is available. For example, if the IBCLC is only at the hospital Monday through Friday and you give birth on the weekend, you may never see the lactation consultant. If the lactation consultant tries to see all the mothers, she may seem abrupt or like her mind is already on the next patient.

We actually know how many lactation consultants are necessary to provide good care. According to Mannel and Mannel (2006) the optimal staffing for IBCLCs is one full-time equivalent (FTE) per 783 births, with one FTE for every 235 infants admits. For outpatient care, there should be one FTE for every 1,292 mother–infant pairs.

Unfortunately, many hospitals do not have this level of staffing. In our informal survey of 361 mothers, 38% indicated that they did not see a lactation consultant in the hospital at all. Sixty-six percent said that someone did watch them breastfeed, but only 40% said that someone made sure that their babies were drinking milk before they were discharged. That's a large percentage of mothers and babies not receiving good care.

If hospital lactation support is not available, all is not lost. If you didn't get hospital support and are struggling, I hope you take heart from these survey results. Even though many of the women in my survey did not have good hospital lactation support, almost all were able to successfully breastfeed; 79% exclusively breastfed, and 56% exclusively breastfed until their babies started solids, which is much higher than the U.S. average (Centers for Disease Control and Prevention, 2020a).

Mothers can also struggle to get connected with support once they leave the hospital. Lack of postpartum support can be a perennial problem, as this mother described:

> The hospital did not set up a follow-up appointment. I had to figure that out. They also did not call to follow up on progress. Both would have gone a long way. I waited too long to get help because I had no guidance/outreach/support from my providers.

If you run into something similar, I'd urge you to be proactive in getting help. If there's no help in your community, see if there's some help in a nearby town. You can also find support online. Don't wait because it's always better to address problems sooner rather than later. Look up breastfeeding peer support programs such as La Leche League, Baby Cafes, Breastfeeding USA, and WIC (United States); La Leche League, Canada (each province has its own breastfeeding support organization); La Leche League, Breastfeeding Network, Nursing Mothers' Association, or National Childbirth Trust (United Kingdom); and the Australian Breastfeeding Association.

PHYSICIAN OR MIDWIFE SUPPORT

Midwives and physicians can be great sources of support or part of the problem. Midwives generally have some training in breastfeeding, but physicians do not unless they have sought it out themselves. This isn't surprising because most medical training programs do not cover it at all. As someone who has trained many pediatric residents, I can tell you that most of them knew little about breastfeeding, but people expect them to know. They're in a tough position. When physicians have extra training, their assistance is often outstanding.

My pediatrician is a lactation consultant whose support was monumental when my newborn was rapidly losing weight.

It is also helpful when physicians refer you to a lactation consultant or have one on staff. . . . Our pediatrician's office has a CLC [certified lactation counselor] on staff so I was able to ask her a few questions that came up.

This mother received support from her pediatrician, a breastfeeding class, and from other mothers:

We have an amazing pediatrician. I also studied breastfeeding before my first and went to nursing groups when she was born. Those moms helped me with their own trial and error, so I always try to help new moms with good info as well.

The most problematic group, in my view, are the physicians who don't know anything about breastfeeding but think that they do. This group never refers. For these providers, supplementation and weaning are the answers to every problem. It can be a jolt to realize that your health care provider does not have all the answers, but when you recognize this, it allows you to trust your gut. If something doesn't feel right, *get a second opinion*. If you recognize your health care providers' limitations, you can seek the support you need from other sources. It's really okay to do that. For most new mothers, breastfeeding support will probably not come from physicians unless they have received outside training. That may change at some point, but we're not there yet.

Providers' Attitude About Breastfeeding

Your provider's attitude about breastfeeding can influence your care in ways that you might never expect. Confidence is so important in breastfeeding support. Breastfeeding-medicine specialist Dr. Tina Smillie says we must "ooze confidence" that breastfeeding will work. If providers lack confidence, mothers pick it up. A negative attitude can creep out in a dozen subtle ways: a raised brow, lack of eye contact, a sigh.

One study of pediatricians examined changes in their breastfeeding recommendations and beliefs from 1995 to 2014 (Feldman-Winter et al., 2017). On the plus side, pediatricians were more likely to recommend exclusive breastfeeding and a Day 5 visit than in 1995. Unfortunately, these same pediatricians were less likely to believe that mothers could successfully breastfeed or that breastfeeding risks outweighed the benefits. Only 47% referred mothers to community support groups, and pediatricians felt less confident that they could manage breastfeeding problems.

These findings are ominous. Of all health care providers, pediatricians are the ones American mothers are most likely to turn to. These doctors are saying all the politically correct things—"Yes, breast is best," "Yes, mothers should exclusively breastfeed," and "Yes, their hospitals should be baby-friendly"—yet their attitude often communicated something else.

The second study focused on how to educate providers about breastfeeding and included Swedish midwives and health visitors (Ekstrom & Thorstensson, 2015). Providers received one of two training types: information only or information plus a chance to process their own breastfeeding experiences. The researchers then randomly assigned 585 mothers to those providers for care. The mothers did not know which type of training their providers had received, but the effects of that training were far-reaching.

Mothers in the information-and-processing group initiated breastfeeding earlier, breastfed more frequently during the first 24 hours, and used formula less often in the hospital and after discharge. After discharge, the mothers were more satisfied; had fewer breastfeeding problems, such as insufficient milk; and breastfed longer. They also felt more positively about their babies than mothers in the information-only group. The differences were still apparent at 1 year postpartum. Mothers in the information-and-processing group believed that they received more support, even from providers who were not in the study, than mothers in the information-only group.

These findings highlight a couple of important things. First, information only is not a great way to train people to provide breastfeeding support, but it is the way that we tend to do it. Second, if providers have had negative breastfeeding experiences, or know someone who has, it leaks into their care until they have a chance to process it. If someone is negative with you, it may have more to do with their issues than yours.

Some Other Cautions in Terms of Selecting a Provider

It's in your best interest to educate yourself but also consider how you are treated. Did the provider listen respectfully to your concerns, or did they blow you off? Mothers often know something is wrong before providers do, and wise providers listen to mothers. I'd urge you to avoid the arrogant ones because they may miss something important and generally undermine you.

Another red flag is seeing materials from formula companies in their offices or waiting rooms: pens, notepads, clocks, or information booklets. Although formula can be necessary, formula companies have a vested interest in making breastfeeding fail. They will give you some good information while planting seeds of doubt ("Here's a coupon just in case things don't work out"). Health care as a whole is paying more attention to industry sponsorship and conflict of interest, yet some physicians still get their "breastfeeding" training from conferences sponsored by formula companies. If you see these signs, know that you will most likely not get good breastfeeding advice from that physician. Physicians do not have to rely on free-bies from the formula companies. There are many low-cost, non-commercially sponsored alternatives that will have more accurate information.

LACTATION CONSULTANTS AND SPECIALISTS

Lactation specialists include a wide range of professionals and vol-unteers who work with new mothers. All specialists have hours of training and may or may not be professionals in other fields, such as nursing, medicine, speech and language, physical therapy, or psy-chology. Education and credentials are important, but they are not the only things. Some people are highly educated but are terrible clinicians. Even great clinicians don't necessarily click with every mother. Shop around, talk with mothers, and find someone you'd like to work with. When you interact with them, do you feel empowered or demoralized? The goal is to help you reach your breastfeeding goals, not theirs. It can feel like a lot to sort through all these options in the early days. This is one area where your partner or support person can really help by identifying resources in your community.

Sorting Through Credentials

So many credentials have sprouted up over the past few years that it can be confusing to know which one is best. The IBCLC is the gold standard for lactation care. However, as with anything involving human beings, there is a huge variation in knowledge and clinical skills. The U.S. Lactation Consultant Association (2020) described the range of support available:

> Breastfeeding support ranges from basic encouragement and emotional support to guidance and assistance with complex

clinical situations, all of which play a vital role in providing care to families. The varied categories of lactation care providers differ greatly in terms of training and experience. Recognizing these differences can be confusing to both families as well as allied healthcare team members.

You may encounter an IBCLC or certified lactation counselor (CLC). Other credentials include certified breastfeeding educators (CBE), certified lactation specialist (CLS), or baby café breastfeeding counselors (BCBC). Feel free to ask about their training and qualifications. Your pediatrician may also have an IBCLC or CLC on staff, which is, in my view, ideal.

The U.S. Lactation Consultant Association developed a chart summarizing different categories of lactation specialists, their education, and their training (see Table 12.1). Although training and education are important, they are not everything; some of the best and most experienced clinicians I know are volunteers, not IBCLCs.

For countries outside the United States, a midwife is often the one who provides care, and a home visitor checks on families after they leave the hospital. These providers may or may not have breastfeeding credentials. Some mothers find that hospital lactation support is limited, community lactation support is more helpful:

> I started with a nipple shield and did not get much help in hospital regarding breastfeeding. I struggled with nurses trying to help. I saw a lactation specialist the last day right before discharge even though she was requested much sooner. She was not very helpful but felt I had sort of figured it out enough on my own to be confident at home. . . . Once I was home, I contacted local lactation specialist group (Berkshire Nursing Families) and did so much better and had so much more confidence. They told me to use the nipple shield if that's what works and then worked with me to eventually wean off of it.

TABLE 12.1. Who's Who? An At-a-Glance Look at Lactation Support in the United States

Lactation provider category	Prerequisites	Training required	Scope of practice
International Board Certified Lactation Consultant (IBCLC)	Recognized health professional or satisfactory completion of college-level health sciences coursework	• 90 hours of lactation-specific education • College-level science courses • 300–1,000 clinical practice hours • Successful completion of a criterion-referenced exam offered by an independent international board of examiners	Provide professional, evidence-based, clinical lactation management; educate families, health professionals, and others about human lactation
Counselor/Educator (Certified Lactation Counselor, Breastfeeding Educator, etc.)	N/A	• 20–120 hours of classroom training • Often includes a written exam or certification offered by the training organization	Provide education and guidance for families on basic breast-feeding issues
Peer supporter (La Leche League, Breastfeeding USA, WIC peer counselor, Nursing Mothers' Association, Breastfeeding Network)	Personal breastfeeding experience	• 18–50 hours of classroom training/independent study • Mentoring by experienced volunteers	Provide breastfeeding information, encouragement, and support to those in their community

Note. From *Who's Who? An At-a-Glance Look at Lactation Support in the United States*, by the United States Lactation Consultant Association, 2020 (https://uslca.org/wp-content/uploads/2019/07/Whos-Who-August-2020.pdf). Copyright 2020 by USLCA. Reprinted with permission.

This mother shared a similar story and indicated that the combination of a lactation consultant and breastfeeding support group worked best for her. She did not receive support from physicians.

> Without my lactation consultant and a breastfeeding support group, I would not have been as successful. My OB and pediatrician were little help in the breastfeeding department. The nurses and lactation consultants made the difference.

Another mother benefitted from both a breastfeeding class and her lactation consultant:

> I took a breastfeeding class at the hospital while still pregnant. That, along with talking to my LC after my baby was born, was the most helpful resource I had.

This mother, however, reported that her lactation consultant made her feel bad because she wanted to use a pacifier. She made breastfeeding work, but she did it in a way that many lactation consultants would not recommend:

> My daughter has a very strong suck and we struggled with pain. We really wanted to use a pacifier to help when she just wanted to suck, but not eat. We received a lot of criticism because of that from the lactation consultant. We ultimately used a pacifier and supplemented with bottles (due to weight loss) and we are still successful with breastfeeding. I felt a lot of shame at first because of our decision to use the pacifier because of the pressure from the lactation consultant.

Scope of Practice

A particularly thorny issue in lactation care is the scope of practice. Scope of practice refers to how much the person you are consulting with can do when helping you. For example, none of the professionals or volunteers are allowed to make medical diagnoses unless they are also physicians, midwives, or nurse practitioners. However, IBCLCs can say that something is consistent with X, Y, Z conditions. Even volunteer peer counselors can say something like "that looks like thrush" or "that sounds like mastitis" and refer you to your health care provider. It is within their scope of practice to suggest that a mother follow up on a particular symptom or talk to pediatrician about something they've observed. That is ethical; making a diagnosis is not.

CONCLUSION

Professional support can come from the hospital (either inpatient or outpatient care) or in the community. Breastfeeding supporters can include health care providers or those with specialized lactation credentials. When you decide on a care provider, pay attention to both their knowledge and how you feel. If you are not feeling heard, find another provider. There are many choices available, and some lactation consultants are offering their services via Zoom. Some providers are covered by health insurance, and some are private pay. Volunteer peer supporters offer their services for free. As a general rule, it's good to inquire about price before you begin services. The most important goal with any type of support is to feel empowered to reach your breastfeeding goals. If you do not feel that way, talk to someone else. You're the mother. This is your decision.

CHAPTER 13

WHAT POSTPARTUM SUPPORT COULD BE

Is ours not a strange culture that focuses so much attention on childbirth—virtually all of it based on anxiety and fear— and so little on the crucial time after birth, when patterns are established that will affect the individual and the family for decades?

—Suzanne Arms

In many Western countries, mothers disappear after birth as everyone's focus now shifts to the baby. It's been called the "reverse Cinderella." You went from pregnant princess to postpartum peasant with a wave of your obstetrician's wand. When you were pregnant, people held doors for you, and they asked how you felt. People saw you, and they cared.

Since you had your baby, no one asks about you anymore. When people come over, who do they want to see? This shocking transition happens without warning. You have been through a major event, and although most mothers and babies survive birth, you are acutely aware that you walked on the knife-edge of life and death. No matter how it happened, it's a big deal, but mothers are treated as if it's not. It doesn't have to be this way.

Mothers in Western (particularly American) culture falsely compare themselves to the apocryphal mother in the field who has a baby, puts it on her back, and gets right back to work. They think that's what they should do too. Does this happen in some poorer countries? Yes, sometimes. Is it ideal? Definitely not.

One of the best analyses of postpartum support across cultures came from two anthropologists in the 1980s called Stern and Kruckman (1983). They found that in some cultures, rates of postpartum depression were low. Even the baby blues, which are ubiquitous in Western cultures (typically 55%–85% of new mothers), were exceptionally low. Stern and Kruckman posited that something about these cultures was protecting the mental health of new mothers, so they examined the postpartum rituals from a wide range of cultures. They noted that there were five social structures that protected the mental health of new mothers. The specific activities within these structures varied by culture. Many of these countries were lower income, yet their care for new mothers far exceeded the efforts of more affluent nations. As for the mother in the field, women in these cultures would be exceedingly sad. That's not the ideal to aim for; it's a sign of extreme deprivation.

SOCIAL STRUCTURES THAT PROTECT NEW MOTHERS

Although the specific actions differ from culture to culture, these structures served the same purpose of supporting mothers and babies through a vulnerable time.

A Distinct Postpartum Period

In cultures with low rates of postpartum mental illness, postpartum is recognized as a distinct time from normal life. Mothers are supposed to recuperate, their activities are limited, and their female relatives take care of them. In colonial America, postpartum was called the "lying-in" period. This period functioned as a time of apprenticeship, when more experienced mothers mentored the new mother. Forty days were commonly marked as the postpartum period in Judaism, Christianity, and Islam. This is similar to the 40-day period in Latin America, *la cuarantena* ("the quarantine") and "doing the month" in China (Eberhard-Gran et al., 2010).

Protective Measures Reflecting the New Mother's Vulnerability

During the postpartum period, new mothers are recognized as being especially vulnerable. Rituals protected the mother and set aside this time as distinct from normal life. Food also plays a role in this structure. For example, in China, mothers must have a special hot postpartum tea and avoid cold foods and drinks. (Avoiding cold foods is pretty common in Chinese medicine, in general. When I was teaching at a hospital in China, even milk is served piping hot.) Postpartum porridge was common in the Middle Ages as something that guests would bring that would protect mother and child (Eberhard-Gran et al., 2010).

Other protective measures included the wrapping of mothers' head or abdomen. From a modern perspective, wrapping the abdomen helps the uterus contract. Warmth increases mothers' oxytocin (Uvnäs Moberg, 2013). Limiting visitors also protects new mothers. During COVID-19, limiting visitation actually protected the mother while she was in the hospital. Visits can be exhausting and make it difficult to get breastfeeding off to a good start. Postpartum doula Salle Webber (2012) described the care that mothers need in the *Gentle Art of Newborn Family Care*:

> In traditional and tribal cultures, mother and child are cared for, sheltered, and protected for up to 40 days after birth. Women

of the community attend to their personal needs, and care for the home and family. Generally, the mother and infant don't leave home during that time. It is understood that this period is delicate, baby's life is tenuous, and the mother needs to rebuild her strength to feed and care for her child in the years ahead.

To the tribe, each life is valuable, and they worked together to provide the best possible outcome, knowing that life can slip away quickly. With our modern medical facilities, we often fail to recall what a tremendous miracle it is to undergo a pregnancy and childbirth, and to raise a child. We expect successful outcomes, yet the possibilities of complications are vast, as our foremothers knew all too well. It is prudent to treat the postpartum weeks in a tender and careful way, as an investment in the long-term health and well-being of mother and child. (pp. 25–26)

Social Seclusion and Mandated Rest

Related to the concept of vulnerability are the widespread practices of social seclusion for new mothers. During this time, she is supposed to rest and restrict normal activities. In our busy culture, we fight against this. Even the Puritans, who expected people to work hard, didn't expect new mothers to immediately resume work. Why? Because it increased the risk of death for mothers and babies. So if the founders of the Protestant Work Ethic gave new mothers a lying-in period, shouldn't we?

In the Punjab, women are secluded from everyone but female relatives and the midwife for 5 days, after which there is a "stepping-out" ceremony for the mother and baby. In some cultures, the time of seclusion can be up to 3 months. Seclusion and rest also allow mothers to recover, promote breastfeeding, and limit their normal activities. In Nigeria, women and infants are isolated in a "fattening room," where the mother's duty, for 2 or 3 months postpartum, is to gain weight, sleep, and care for her infant (Eberhard-Gran et al., 2010).

Functional Assistance

To ensure that women are getting the rest they need, they must be relieved of their normal workload. Functional assistance involves care of older children, household help, and personal attendance during labor. In many cultures, women return to their families' homes to ensure that this type of assistance is available. In Germany, *Wochenbett* (weeks in bed) means that women should not only rest but stay in bed during the postpartum period (Eberhard-Gran et al., 2010). Salle Webber said that a doctor in her community of Santa Cruz, California, prescribes 2 weeks in bed, 2 weeks on the bed, and 2 weeks near the bed for her new mothers (Webber, 2012). Taking time to rest doesn't make you weak; it means that you're doing what you need to do to recover from creating a tiny human.

Social Recognition of Her New Role and Status

Another structure includes rituals that provide personal attention to the mother and recognizing her new status through social rituals and gifts. For example, in Punjabi culture, there is the ritual stepping-out ceremony, ritual bathing and hair washing performed by the midwife, and a ceremonial meal prepared by a brahmin. When she returns to her husband's family, she brings gifts she has received for herself and her baby.

Ritual bathing, washing of hair, massage, binding of the abdomen, and other types of personal care are also prominent in the postpartum rituals of rural Guatemala, Mayan women in the Yucatan, and Latinas both in the United States and Mexico. Here is a description of one of these recognition rituals performed by the Chagga people of Uganda. This is an older example, but it remains one of my favorites:

> Three months after the birth of her child, the Chagga woman's head is shaved and crowned with a bead tiara, she is robed in

an ancient skin garment worked with beads, a staff such as the elders carry is put in her hand, and she emerges from her hut for her first public appearance with her baby. Proceeding slowly toward the market, they are greeted with songs such as are sung to warriors returning from battle. She and her baby have survived the weeks of danger. The child is no longer vulnerable, but a baby who has learned what love means, has smiled its first smiles and is now ready to learn about the bright, loud world outside. (Dunham, 1992, p. 148)

THE RISE OF THE POSTPARTUM DOULA

I've been encouraged to see a wonderful change in the birth industry: the rise of the postpartum doula. Although postpartum doulas have been around for decades, they were not mainstream until recently as more people recognize their benefits. A postpartum doula is someone who takes care of the household so mothers can get the rest they need. They may grocery shop, start dinner, provide company and emotional support, offer basic breastfeeding support, and can be a bridge to other resources in the community (Webber, 2012).

Why Doulas Are Important

The word *doula* is Greek for "servant" and is a term that Dana Raphael first used in her classic book, *The Tender Gift* (Raphael, 1955). Like labor-support doulas, postpartum doulas grew organically from a need in their communities. My friend Salle Webber became a postpartum doula before there was even a name for it. She started by helping a friend who had recently given birth, which led to other opportunities, including referrals from a midwife practice whose patients needed someone who could help them postpartum. Her business grew from there.

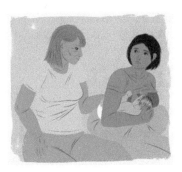

Postpartum doulas provide practical assistance and emotional support.

I first ran across Salle Webber when I read an article she'd written for a little magazine called *The Doula*, which I also wrote for. It shows what good postpartum support could look like for you.

In my work as a Doula, my focus is on the mother. I want to provide whatever it is that she needs to feel comfortable, nourished, relaxed, and appreciated: to facilitate a harmonious transition for both mother and child in those profound first days and weeks after birth. A mother needs someone who cares about how many times the baby woke to nurse in the night, how many diapers were changed, how her breasts are feeling. She may need her back massaged, or her sheets changed, or she may need someone to provide an abundant supply of water or tea, salads readymade in the refrigerator, a bowl of cut-up fruit. She needs to be able to complain about how little her mate understands what she's going through, and perhaps, some gentle reminders of all the contributions he has made. She needs someone to hold the baby so she can take a shower or even go to the bathroom; someone to answer the phone when she's napping; someone to water her plants or garden, to clean the kitchen and bathroom, to keep up on the family's laundry. She may have many questions and concerns that only an experienced mother can understand. She needs patience and kind words and a clean and calm environment. (Webber, 1992, p. 17)

Why Postpartum Doulas Are Good for You

The importance of postpartum doulas is not just anecdote. We now have some studies showing that they help women, especially in vulnerable situations. For example, a recent qualitative study of 13 disadvantaged mothers and 19 volunteer doulas in the United Kingdom emphasized the importance of doula support to mothers' health and well-being (McLeish & Redshaw, 2019). In this study, volunteer doulas reduced anxiety, unhappiness, and stress, and increased mothers' self-esteem and self-efficacy. Doulas helped mothers feel more skillful, make the best use of available maternity services, and build ties to support community organizations. The mothers valued the doula's support, and it helped them improve in their parenting skills and confidence. Breastfeeding was not specifically mentioned, but there was a positive effect on mothers' mental health.

Another study was a randomized trial with low-income African American mothers (Edwards et al., 2013). Doula care from pregnancy to 3 months postpartum increased breastfeeding rates. Mothers in the doula group had higher rates of breastfeeding initiation, breastfed longer than 6 weeks, and waited longer before introducing solids. The authors concluded that doulas likely succeeded because of the relationship with the mother based on shared culture, prenatal home visiting, and the doula's presence at birth, which got breastfeeding off to a good start.

These mothers in my survey also described how their post-partum doula helped them breastfeed:

> I hired a very pro-breastfeeding doula for the birth who stayed to help make sure my baby was feeding properly and who gave me confidence in my abilities to breastfeed.

> My oldest slept so much in the hospital that he hardly nursed. I did see a lactation consultant who gave me good advice. My youngest nursed right away, no difficulties. My doula friend was there and made sure he latched properly.

Doula care even helps mothers at high-risk for depression. Thirty-nine mothers with depressive symptoms were randomized to receive either postpartum doula care or follow-up phone calls (Gjerdingen et al., 2013). At the beginning of the study, more women in the doula group had a history of depression. At 6 months post-partum, more women in the doula group were depressed but were receiving treatment for depression. That may not sound like a positive finding, but mothers in the doula group were happy with the care and more satisfied than mothers who received telephone follow-up. The higher number of depressed women in the doula group could be a sur-veillance effect, where depression was identified because there was a doula in the home. Women without doulas may have had lower rates of depression because their depression was not identified.

The Seven Sisters Approach

If you cannot afford a doula, or there is not one available in your community, an alternative is the Seven Sisters method popularized by Michelle Peterson (2016). In her book, *Seven Sisters for Seven Days*, she recommends that women ask for postpartum help rather than baby gifts. *Seven Sisters* provides a structure that helps your friends help you; friends sign up for a specific day of the week and commit to providing care on that day for the next few weeks. One person could pick up groceries, another could do laundry or some light housework, still another could bring a meal. Peterson recommends that friends pick a task that they enjoy doing for their day. If it's laundry, they do laundry. If it's cooking, that's what they do. Her book offers specific suggestions, including sample letters to send to friends. This can be an inexpensive alternative to doula care.

Postpartum Care, Not Sleep Training

A concerning trend has been for some postpartum doulas to also offer sleep-training services, where they sleep train your baby for you. Unfortunately, this is a popular service, and I think a lot of parents feel peer-pressured into asking for it (thinking it's just part of baby care). However, if you want to be able to meet your breastfeeding goals, I'd recommend avoiding this. It's similar to the old concept of the "baby nurse" that promoted a lot of mother–infant separation. Although it might be tempting to avoid nighttime feeds, that strategy increases your risk for both breastfeeding problems and depression (Dørheim et al., 2009a; Kendall-Tackett et al., 2011; Kendall-Tackett, Cong, et al., 2018). If you hire a postpartum doula, find out what types of services they offer so that you will be on the same page in terms of what you want and so that you won't feel pressured into getting services you don't want. In can be hard to advocate for yourself in the heat of the moment. Better to have this discussion before you need services.

CONCLUSION

Although our culture lacks supportive postpartum rituals, the work of individuals, such as doulas, can make a significant difference. Many are surprised that this decidedly low-tech intervention can work, yet this is perhaps the most important lesson we can learn from the cultures that Stern and Kruckman described. We know what we need to do to help mothers successfully transition to new motherhood. I truly hope that this has given you "permission" to take the time you need to recover and get breastfeeding off to a good start. It is ethnocentric to think that the typical Western way is always the best, when it clearly isn't. I'd like to close this chapter with another lovely quote from Salle Webber's (2012) *Gentle Art of Newborn Family Care*:

> I sometimes suggest the parents take a nap together when I'm available for infant care or go for a short walk or out to lunch. This is a tender, wonderful, and difficult time for these individuals. No experience can really prepare a person for parenthood, and it comes on full force. Helping them ease into these new roles is an act of kindness. We can provide the parents with short breaks, or respite from the non-stop responsibility of newborn care—a chance to catch their breath, to regroup before continuing on. (p. 12)

VI

CARING FOR YOUR MENTAL HEALTH

INTRODUCTION: CARING FOR YOUR MENTAL HEALTH

In the early days of motherhood, it's easy to lose yourself. Your baby needs care, but so do you. Caring for your mental health is critical and will make it easier for you to meet the challenges of this time, as lactation consultant Chris Auer (2021) described, "When all is dark . . . there is guilt over not feeling enthralled with her newborn, it's hard for a mom . . . to envision that she will feel herself again" (p. 67).

Unfortunately, some mothers become depressed, anxious, or have symptoms of posttraumatic stress disorder (PTSD). The rates of postpartum depression range from 15% to 25% of new mothers, but that percentage increases with higher-risk groups (Kendall-Tackett, 2017). Data on mothers who are racial/ethnic minorities in the United States show higher rates for American Indians or Alaska Natives (Bauman et al., 2020). Data on postpartum sexual minorities are sparse, but the rate is also likely higher.

Postpartum depression, anxiety, and PTSD fall under the general title of postpartum mood and anxiety disorders. These conditions are predictable and based on risk factors. As a breastfeeding mother, your risk is lower, but you are still susceptible.

CHAPTER 14

POSTPARTUM MOOD DISORDERS AND D-MER

RISK FACTORS FOR POSTPARTUM DEPRESSION, ANXIETY, AND PTSD

There are many things that make mothers vulnerable to postpartum disorders. Here are some of the most common (Kendall-Tackett, 2007, 2017):

- *Ongoing stress.* If you have chronic stress, you are more vulnerable to postpartum depression, anxiety, and posttraumatic stress disorder (PTSD) because stress increases inflammation (see Chapter 4).
- *Pain.* Pain is a potent trigger for depression because your body thinks it's under attack and increases inflammation. If you have pain, we need to find out why and address it.
- *History of affective disorders.* If you've had previous depression, anxiety, or PTSD, you are at increased risk of recurrence, but it is not inevitable.
- *History of trauma.* Many new mothers have a history of trauma that increases risk for a variety of reasons, including increasing chronic inflammation (Danese et al., 2009; Rich-Edwards et al., 2010).

- *Traumatic birth.* Your birth experience can also increase your risk for depression, anxiety, and PTSD.
- *Infertility or previous infant loss.* Both are highly stressful, can lead to high-intervention births, and shape your views about yourself as a mother. You may have also experienced prior infant loss and have unresolved grief.
- *Cultural considerations.* Although we are in the early stages of research on this topic, preliminary evidence suggests that women from marginalized groups have a higher risk for depression and other disorders (Centers for Disease Control and Prevention, 2020b). However, even when there is marginalization, strong relationships within families or their community buffers many of these effects.

Following is a brief summary of depression, anxiety, and PTSD. I also describe postpartum psychosis, which happens to one in 1,000 mothers. Finally, I describe a condition specific to breastfeeding: dysphoric milk-ejection reflex (D-MER).

POSTPARTUM DEPRESSION

Postpartum depression (PPD) is depression that develops in the first 12 months after birth. When diagnosing PPD, practitioners use the criteria for major depressive disorder in the fifth edition of the *Diagnostic and Statistical Manual of Mental Disorders* (DSM-5; American Psychiatric Association, 2013). Those symptoms include feelings of sadness, not enjoying even things you used to like to do, trouble going to and staying asleep, feeling foggy, trouble concentrating, or feeling angry. You may believe that you will never be a good-enough mother (Centers for Disease Control and Prevention, 2020b). If these symptoms persist for 2 weeks or longer, follow up with your health care provider or contact Postpartum Support International (https://www.postpartum.net). In the *DSM-5*, there is no specific category for PPD. If symptoms occur in the first 4 weeks after birth, the practitioner can add "with postpartum onset" to the appropriate diagnosis. The diagnostic criteria for various conditions in the *DSM* are helpful. However, defining "postpartum" as the first 4 weeks is odd. Even obstetricians say 6 weeks. It's actually the research literature that specifies 1 year postpartum. That definition makes sense to anyone who works with new families because symptoms may not appear right away and, in some cases, will not manifest for months.

How Depression Influences Breastfeeding

Hundreds of studies have documented the harmful effects of parents' depression on their children. Researchers have tried to figure out why these effects occur. When it comes down to it, depression in mothers (and fathers) is harmful to children because it negatively affects the way they interact with their children (Oddy et al., 2010; Strathearn et al., 2009). Most of the research has been done with mothers, but I want to acknowledge that we also see this in fathers. Mothers who are depressed tend to interact in one of two ways: They either disengage from their babies or they are angry and intrusive. Both styles can lead to negative effects (Diego et al., 2006).

Of the hundreds of studies on the harmful effects of maternal depression on babies, only one included feeding method (Jones et al., 2004). This study included four groups: breastfeeding mothers who were either depressed or nondepressed and formula-feeding mothers who were either depressed or nondepressed. The researchers examined babies' electroencephalogram (EEG; brain-wave) patterns and looked for an abnormal pattern you see in chronically depressed adults. The depressed, formula-feeding mothers had babies with the abnormal EEG pattern, but the babies of the depressed, breastfeeding mothers had normal EEG patterns. In other words, *breastfeeding protected those babies from the harmful effects of their mothers' depression.* Why? Because the depressed, breastfeeding mothers could not disengage from their babies. They looked at, touched, and talked to their babies more than the depressed, formula-feeding mothers. It may not have been as much as they would normally do, but it was enough to protect their babies. If you are depressed and formula-feeding, you can make a conscious effort to interact with your baby, which helps, but with breastfeeding, those types of interactions are built into the system (Kendall-Tackett, 2017).

POSTPARTUM ANXIETY

Postpartum anxiety takes many forms. There is generalized anxiety disorder, where many things make you anxious and you worry about everything, or agoraphobia, where you are afraid to leave your home. Or you may have postpartum obsessive–compulsive disorder (OCD).

Anxiety and Breastfeeding

As a lactation consultant, I've worked with several mothers who had severe anxiety. They were anxious about their milk supply and their babies' weight, even when there was no actual problem. If you feel this way, information is power. How is your baby's weight? That is the gold standard. If weighing reassures you, there's no harm in it. If constant weight checks make you more anxious, however, try doing it less often as long as there is not a specific health issue where tracking is necessary. Mindfulness can also help. I'd recommend Dr. Diane Sanford's (2019) book, *Stress Less, Live Better: For Pregnancy, Postpartum, and Early Motherhood.*

Anxiety can also influence pumping and storing milk. One mother I saw at 2 weeks postpartum had a freezer full of milk. She was scared to death that she would run out. The extra pumping she was doing doubled her workload, and it would be hard to keep up that pace for any length of time. The same applies to "triple feeding" when you feed at the breast, pump, and then feed your baby with a bottle. Yes, this strategy can help for a short time *when there is a documented case of low milk supply*. Unfortunately, anxious mothers might do this "just in case."

Postpartum OCD

OCD is an anxiety disorder that can occur alone or with postpartum depression and is characterized by recurrent, unwelcome thoughts, or doubt (Abramowitz et al., 2003). One of the most difficult manifestations of OCD is when mothers have persistent thoughts of infant harm, as one mother described in *Depression in New Mothers*:

> If I was ironing, I'd be terrified that the baby would be burned. Even if he was upstairs asleep in his bed. Then I would start to analyze my thoughts. "Am I thinking he'd be burned because I wanted him to be burned?" I was also scared of knives . . . I didn't want to do these things. I couldn't understand why I was thinking this way. . . . These thoughts happened every day, all the time. (Kendall-Tackett, 2017, p.19)

Thoughts about infant harm are serious, and you should pay attention to them, but actual harm is rare. So how can you tell when it's random thoughts versus thoughts that increase the risk of harm? Mothers with OCD are horrified and feel guilty that they've had these awful thoughts. Mothers at risk for infant harm don't feel guilty and may even feel justified (Abramowitz et al., 2003; Speisman et al., 2011), especially if they are in the throes of postpartum psychosis.

If you are isolated and feel like you might harm your infant, put them in a safe place and walk away. I've talked with mothers over the years who have gotten to that point. It's a sign that you need some help, even if it's just someone to give you a break during the day. Find a mother's group, take a daily walk outside with your baby, call a friend, or hire a teenager to help in the afternoon. These are all important parts of taking care of yourself and your baby.

PTSD

PTSD is a syndrome that occurs in response to traumatic events. To be diagnosed with PTSD, you much meet the full set of criteria. First, the event needs to rise to a certain threshold of severity. The current criteria are that the event needs to include death or threatened death, actual or threatened serious injury, or actual or threatened sexual violation. You need symptoms in four clusters, and the symptoms have had to continue for at least 1 month, with significant impairment in your daily life (American Psychiatric Association, 2013). Trauma is such an important topic that both Chapters 15 and 16 focus on it. I discuss it only briefly here.

If you've experienced trauma, you might feel disconnected from others, including your baby. If you were separated, you may feel that you don't even "know" them. If you are feeling detached, find ways to reconnect. Wear your baby, hang out together, do skin-to-skin, take your baby to bed for a couple of days. Enlist whatever help you need to make that happen, whether it's family, friends, or a postpartum doula.

WHAT YOU CAN DO ABOUT PPD, ANXIETY, AND PTSD

Treatment of postpartum mood disorders and PTSD can involve complementary and integrative modalities, along with psychotherapy and medications. In this section, I include a brief overview of various treatments for postpartum depression, anxiety, and some trauma symptoms. Trauma treatment is more specialized. If you would like more detail about your options for trauma care, a great resource is the National Center for PTSD. The site is set up for combat veterans, but it has great content for anyone who has experienced trauma.

Complementary and Integrative Treatments

Many mothers prefer complementary and integrative treatments for mood disorders and PTSD. These can be combined with medications and psychotherapy or can be used separately. If you want to use these modalities, I suggest that you make a plan for what you want to do. It helps if you write it down and discuss it with your partner, friend, or trusted provider. The more specific you are, the more likely you will be to succeed. It could look something like this:

Exercise three times a week. Walk in the park for 30 minutes. Attend mother–baby yoga once a week.

Take 1,000 mg of EPA (eicosapentaenoic acid) every day.

Next, you should monitor your progress by writing down each activity as you do it, such as when you exercise. Depression, in particular, can make you feel like not doing anything, so it's important for you to keep track to make sure you are doing it. Think about how you will record your progress using an app, a journal, calendar, or notebook.

Finally, take a self-assessment for depression, anxiety, or PTSD. There are good tools available for free online. Every 3 to 4 weeks, take the assessment again to see if your symptoms have improved. You may need to adjust your plan. Also, empower someone you trust to check on you to see how you are doing. You want to avoid the scenario where you are not improving but keep doing the same thing. Also, someone else may be more objective about how you're doing. That can be important.

To find free self-assessment tools, search online for the following:

- For depression, the Patient Health Questionnaire–2 or the Edinburgh Postnatal Depression Scale
- For anxiety, the Patient Health Questionnaire–4 (this assesses both depression and anxiety)
- For PTSD, the Patient Checklist–5

Information on how to score the assessment tools comes with the questionnaires.

OMEGA-3 FATTY ACIDS

EPA and DHA (docosahexaenoic acid) are long-chain omega-3 fatty acids found in fatty fish, and they have been used to prevent and treat depression. Populations that eat a lot of fish have lower rates of several types of mental illness, including postpartum depression (Hibbeln, 2002). A prospective study in western Norway found that women with low omega-3 levels at 28 weeks' gestation had more depression at 3 months postpartum (Markhus et al., 2013).

A recent review of 18 randomized trials, with 4,052 participants, found that omega-3s were more effective than a placebo in treating depressive symptoms (Mocking et al., 2020). The strongest effect was for postpartum women. Interestingly, omega-3s did not help with depression during pregnancy, but they did lower the risk of preterm birth (Cappelletti et al., 2016; Middleton et al., 2018).

That is especially important for women with depression, anxiety, or PTSD during pregnancy who are at higher risk for preterm birth.

Even in relatively large doses, EPA and DHA are safe during pregnancy and breastfeeding. They also increase resiliency to stress (Dunstan et al., 2004; Grandjean et al., 2001). For pregnant and postpartum women, fish oil capsules are safer than eating fish because of possible contaminants. EPA treats depression, and DHA helps prevent it. EPA specifically lowers inflammation and turns off the stress response (Kiecolt-Glaser et al., 2015; Maes et al., 2000). EPA and DHA have also been combined with medications and make them more effective.

Recommended doses for DHA and EPA are as follows:

- 200 to 400 mg of DHA is the recommended minimum dose, but 800 to 1,000 mg is the typical amount women consume in countries where the population eats a lot of fish (Kendall-Tackett, 2010b).
- 1 gram (1,000 mg) of EPA is the dose used to treat depression.

Read the label of individual fish oil products to see how much DHA and EPA is in one capsule. You may need several capsules to get the recommended dose.

For safe sources of fish oil products, refer to the U.S. Pharmacopeia (https://www.USP.org).

VITAMIN D

Our bodies make vitamin D when they are exposed to sunlight. When people are deficient, they are at risk for a whole host of inflammatory diseases (Wagner et al., 2010). Treating vitamin D deficiency lowers inflammation and helps with depression, anxiety, and PTSD. Vitamin D deficiency is rampant worldwide among pregnant and postpartum women, partly because we spend so much time inside and partly because of our efforts to prevent skin cancer. A prospective study of 796 pregnant women from Perth, Australia, measured vitamin D levels at 18 weeks' gestation and depression at 3 days postpartum (Robinson et al., 2014). The researchers used six items from the Edinburgh Postnatal Depression Scale that measured mood fluctuations, sadness, anxiety, appetite changes, and sleep disturbance. As predicted, women with the lowest vitamin D had the highest depression scores.

Vitamin D is measured with a blood test and needs to be between 30 and 150. Standard recommended supplements are 400 IU/day for adults. However, newer guidelines recommend 4,000 IU/day for pregnant women and 6,400 IU/day for breastfeeding women. Earlier clinical trials demonstrated that these amounts were safe (Wagner et al., 2010).

EXERCISE

Exercise is an effective treatment for depression and is as effective as medication for treating even major depression. Two clinical trials from the Duke University Medical Center compared exercise with sertraline (Zoloft) for adults aged 50 to 80 years (Babyak et al., 2000; Blumenthal et al., 2007). Both studies found that exercise was as effective as sertraline for major depression. A review of 37 studies on exercise and depression found that exercise decreased depressive symptoms (Cooney et al., 2013). It was as effective as psychotherapy in seven trials and as effective as medications in four trials. A review of 13 randomized trials that included a total of 1,734 women found that exercise significantly reduced depressive symptoms in all of the studies (Pritchett et al., 2017). The authors noted that group exercise, participant-chosen exercise, and exercise combined with other interventions can all be effective. Exercise lowers inflammation, and overall fitness level lowers the inflammatory response to stress (Emery et al., 2005; Kiecolt-Glaser et al., 2010; Starkweather, 2007).

Exercise has also been used to treat pregnant and postpartum women. One study randomized mothers to receive a combination of exercise and parenting education (*n* = 62) or education only (*n* = 73) for 8 weeks to treat postpartum depression (Norman et al., 2010). Mothers in education plus exercise group had a 50% drop in their depressive symptoms. They had lower depression scores and higher well-being scores compared with mothers who only received education.

A review article found that leisure-time physical activity decreased depressive symptoms in 17 studies of postpartum depression and exercise (Teychenne & York, 2013). Another review, of 21 studies, found that exercise during pregnancy significantly reduced postpartum depression scores for women who were physically active versus those who were not (Nakamura et al., 2019). Moderate exercise is safe during pregnancy and breastfeeding. It does not decrease milk production or increase lactic acid in the milk (Quinn & Carey, 1999; Su et al., 2007).

The recommended amounts of exercise for depression are as follows.

For mild to moderate depression:

- two or three times per week
- moderate intensity
- 20 to 30 minutes

For major depression:

- three to five times per week
- 60% to 85% maximal capacity
- 45 to 60 minutes

Acupuncture

Acupuncture has been used to treat major depression and PTSD in a number of studies (Kim et al., 2013; Manber et al., 2010). Two clinical trials have shown that acupuncture treated major depression in pregnant women (Manber et al., 2004, 2010). The first trial included 20 women in each group. The percentage of women who recovered from depression was 69% for acupuncture, 47% for sham acupuncture, and 32% for massage (Manber et al., 2004). The second trial included 50 women in each group, and the remission rates were 63% for acupuncture specific to depression, 44% for acupuncture not specific to depression, and 38% for massage (Manber et al., 2010). A recent review of nine studies found that acupuncture reduced depressive symptoms more in intervention than in control groups (Li et al., 2018).

Yoga

Yoga is a newer complementary treatment for postpartum mood disorders and PTSD but has a long history of use in other contexts. In one study, researchers randomized depressed women to either yoga or wait-list conditions. Women in the yoga condition attended classes twice a week for 8 weeks. At the end of the trial, both groups had improved, but women in the yoga group had significantly improved depression, anxiety, and health-related quality of life compared with women in the wait-list group (Buttner et al., 2015).

St. John's Wort

St. John's wort (*Hypericum perforatum*) is the most widely used antidepressant in the world and is generally used for mild to moderate depression (Dugoua et al., 2006). It has been used for major depression, but that is not its standard use. St. John's wort is named so because it blooms near St. John's day (June 24) in the medieval church calendar. "Wort" is the Old English word for medicinal plant. St. John's wort is highly effective in treating depression and is often compared with commercial antidepressants in clinical trials. It was as effective as both sertraline (Zoloft) and paroxetine (Paxil) in two studies, with fewer side effects (Anghelescu et al., 2006; Van Gurp et al., 2002).

The standard dosage is 300 mg three times a day, standardized to 0.3% hypericin. That dose can be doubled if it is not effective (Lawvere & Mahoney, 2005). Used by itself, St. John's wort has an excellent safety record. Very little St. John's wort transfers into milk (Klier et al., 2002). It does interact with several types of medications, however. *Never take St. John's wort with another antidepressant* (Deligiannidis & Freeman, 2010). It also interacts with birth control pills, cyclosporines, antineoplastic agents, HIV medications, and several other classes of medications (Schulz, 2006). Tell your health care provider if you plan to take St. John's wort so that you can do it safely.

Psychotherapy

Psychotherapists or counselors use a variety of techniques or modalities. For postpartum depression, anxiety, and PTSD, two types are commonly used: cognitive behavior therapy (CBT) and interpersonal psychotherapy (IPT). Postpartum Support International (https://www.postpartum.net) has a list of counselors in many communities and also offers telehealth options if there is no local support.

COGNITIVE BEHAVIOR THERAPY

CBT is a highly effective form of psychotherapy that is helpful for depression, anxiety, and trauma. Hundreds of studies show that it's effective, even in clinical trials in which CBT was compared with medications. The premise of CBT is that distortions in people's beliefs about themselves and the world cause depression. People make these assumptions often without being aware that they are doing so. CBT makes those beliefs explicit and then challenges them with the truth. For example, chances are good that you are not the worst mother in the world, even though, at times, you might believe it. By directly addressing these beliefs, symptoms diminish (Rupke et al., 2006).

Recent studies found that CBT is effective for treating postpartum mood disorders and PTSD. Mothers of preterm infants received either a 6- or 9-week course of trauma-focused CBT or one education session (Shaw et al., 2014). At the end of the study, mothers in the CBT group had lower rates of depression, anxiety, and trauma than those in the one-session group. Interestingly, the effects of CBT improved over time. At 6 months postpartum, those in the CBT group had even lower depression, anxiety, and trauma scores than they did at the end of the study.

A recent review of 20 randomized trials, which included data from 3,623 women (Huang et al., 2018), compared CBT treatment for postpartum depression with nontreated women in control groups. CBT effectively lowered women's depression. CBT could be done in person or over the phone. Both were effective.

Interpersonal Psychotherapy

IPT is another frequently used therapy for postpartum depression that can help with anxiety and trauma as well. IPT specifically focuses on social support and helps you identify your key sources of support. How much support do you currently have, and how can you get more support? IPT is effective with mothers even in high-risk situations and has been used to both prevent and treat depression during pregnancy and postpartum (Zlotnick et al., 2006).

A study from China compared IPT to usual care for 180 first-time mothers (Gao et al., 2015). IPT consisted of a 1-hour education session, with one telephone follow-up at 2 weeks postpartum. Those in the IPT group had significantly less depression, more social support, and felt better about themselves as mothers at 6 weeks postpartum compared with those in the usual-care group. A Canadian randomized trial included 241 with postpartum major depression. The women received either standard care or 12 weeks of IPT delivered by a nurse over the phone for 60 minutes once a week (Dennis et al., 2020). By the end of the study, only 11% of women in the IPT group were still depressed compared with 35% in the standard-care group. In addition, women in the IPT group had less anxiety and better partner relationships at all time points. None of the mothers in the IPT group had become depressed again by 36 weeks.

Antidepressants

Antidepressants are a common treatment for perinatal mood disorders, but mothers have complicated feelings about them. Even if antidepressants are prescribed, many mothers resist taking them. The most commonly prescribed antidepressants are from a class called the selective serotonin reuptake inhibitors (SSRIs). These include sertraline (Zoloft), paroxetine (Paxil), fluoxetine (Prozac), citalopram (Celexa), and escitalopram (Lexapro). These increase the neurotransmitter serotonin, which is low in people who are depressed. Another class, serotonin and norepinephrine reuptake inhibitors (SNRIs), increase norepinephrine. These include venlafaxine (Effexor) and duloxetine (Cymbalta). The final group of antidepressants increase dopamine. The most commonly prescribed is bupropion (Wellbutrin), also marketed as Zyban to help people quit smoking. These medications are also used for anxiety and PTSD.

WHAT ABOUT MEDICATIONS IN BREASTMILK?

As a breastfeeding mother, you may worry about passing medication to your baby through your milk. Some practitioners may suggest that you wean "just to be safe," but is it necessary? Usually not. When considering safety, we need to weigh risks associated with medication in breastmilk versus risk associated with not breastfeeding. In most cases, the risk associated with medications in breastmilk is far less compared with risks associated with formula.

> There is only one class of antidepressants that you cannot take while breastfeeding: monoamine oxidase inhibitors (MAOIs).

MEDICATIONS LESS LIKELY TO ENTER MILK

Although most antidepressants are compatible with breastfeeding, some are better than others in terms of the amount that gets into your milk. Ideally, less than 1% of your dose should be in your milk. Information about all medications can be found on the resources I've listed in Exhibit 14.1. Antidepressants with lower transfer rates include sertraline (Zoloft), paroxetine (Paxil), and escitalopram

EXHIBIT 14.1. Resources for Current Medication Recommendations on Medications and Breastfeeding

Medications and Mothers' Milk (Hale, 2021)
Infant Risk Center website: https://infantrisk.com
LactMed online database: https://toxnet.nlm.nih.gov/newtoxnet/lactmed.htm

(Lexapro). If you need another medication besides one of these three, find out how long it takes for it to peak in your plasma, as that is a good proxy for when it peaks in your milk. If you're taking a medication where a higher percentage gets into your milk, find out when the peak is and avoid breastfeeding during that time. Nurse right before you take your medication and then take it. It should clear from your milk in a couple of hours (but check the references in Exhibit 14.1). You may want to have a bottle of pumped milk available in case your baby gets hungry during that time. While avoiding breastfeeding during a medication peak, you don't need to pump your milk to get rid of the medication. The medication gets reabsorbed into your bloodstream and is eliminated from your system.

What to Do if It's Not Working

Medications typically take 4 to 6 weeks to work. While you are waiting for your symptoms to improve, you might consider adding some complementary treatments, such as omega-3 fatty acids and exercise. These work more quickly than antidepressants and increase the effectiveness of medications.

If you decide to go off your medications, talk with your provider first and wean yourself off gradually. Don't do it abruptly or you'll end up in the emergency room.

POSTPARTUM PSYCHOSIS

Postpartum psychosis occurs in 0.1% to 0.2% of all new mothers. Most episodes begin abruptly between Days 3 and 14 postpartum. Bipolar disorder with psychosis is the common condition underlying postpartum psychosis. With this disorder, women may experience hypomanic episodes that include inflated self-esteem, increased talkativeness, decreased sleep, racing thoughts, and increased goal orientation.

Postpartum psychosis can also run in families. Jones and Craddock (2001) examined the 313 deliveries from 152 women who had bipolar disorder. Twenty-six percent had an episode of postpartum psychosis, and 38% of the women had at least one postpartum psychotic episode. Family history of psychosis also increased risk in these women. Twenty-seven of these women had a family history of postpartum psychosis, and 74% developed postpartum psychosis. In contrast, only 30% of these women without a family history had postpartum psychosis.

Postpartum psychosis needs immediate medical intervention because women who have it are at increased risk for postpartum suicide and infanticide. Medication is always necessary. Self-help measures and psychotherapy can support medical interventions but should never be the primary mode of treatment.

Red Flag

If you ever go 2 or 3 days with no sleep, call your health care provider immediately. All of the mothers I've known who had postpartum psychosis were sleepless in the days leading up to their psychotic break.

Summary

If you believe that you have postpartum depression, anxiety, or PTSD, I hope you will avail yourself of one or more of these treatment modalities. You can use complementary modalities, but if your symptoms do not improve, I'd encourage you to reach out to your health care provider. Worst-case scenario is that you do nothing and suffer in silence. Seeking support is not selfish; you and your entire family will benefit, and you will enjoy mothering so much more.

DYSPHORIC MILK-EJECTION REFLEX

D-MER is a condition specific to breastfeeding that can cause mothers a lot of distress, but it is not technically a postpartum mood disorder. With D-MER, mothers experience dysphoria during milk ejection (let-down). They experience a range of negative feelings: dizziness, overwhelming sadness, homesickness, irritation, restlessness, anger, panic, or severe depression or anxiety. In more severe cases, mothers have waves of suicidal ideation and severe depression (see https://www.D-MER.org). There is much we do not know about D-MER, and evidence is anecdotal. There are two published case studies in the literature (Cox, 2010; Heise & Wiessinger, 2011), and the D-MER.org site has many mothers' stories. Incidence is unknown. In the entire population of breastfeeding mothers, it seems relatively rare. However, enough mothers have mentioned it to me that I thought it was important to include.

Symptoms last for the first few minutes of breastfeeding and then subside. Most mothers continue breastfeeding with D-MER, despite these troubling symptoms. For some women, however, the symptoms may be so severe that they stop. D-MER is not postpartum depression or anxiety, but it can co-occur with those conditions, as this mother described:

> It took me quite a while to pick up on the pattern of symptoms I was having because I was simultaneously battling postpartum depression and anxiety. It wasn't until after I had my birth control removed, and I started pumping regularly at work, that I noticed there was a consistent pattern. . . . Every time I pumped or experienced letdown, my symptoms would return with a vengeance. My chest would tighten, my mood would shift to panic and sadness, and I'd sometimes feel quite dizzy. It usually passes within a minute or two of my pumping or nursing session. I experience them more when I pump, and it's been over a year now with no sign of change. (Uvnäs Moberg & Kendall-Tackett, 2018, p. 23)

231

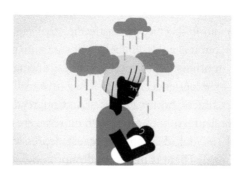

During the first 10 minutes of breastfeeding, women with dysphoric milk-ejection reflex can be overwhelmed with negative feelings.

The symptoms can last anywhere from a few days to several weeks or longer. Some mothers experience symptoms for the entire length of their breastfeeding experiences.

> I had D-MER with all three of my children and symptoms ranged from a general feeling of sadness to suicidal thoughts and to crying. Most of the time it felt like feeling homesick. With my first baby, I noticed symptoms within maybe a week of giving birth, and they lasted about 6 weeks. With my second, I noticed symptoms after my milk surged and they lasted several months. With my third, I pumped antenatally a couple times, and I actually felt it then. It lasted about 4 to 6 weeks with him. Generally, the feelings would wash over me the first few minutes of breastfeeding, and then it would go away within a minute or two of a letdown. (Uvnäs Moberg & Kendall-Tackett, 2018, p. 24)

Dr. Kerstin Uvnäs Moberg and I examined the case reports on the D-MER.org site and applied what we know about the underlying physiology of breastfeeding (Uvnäs Moberg & Kendall-Tackett, 2018). The pattern of symptoms fits the pattern of oxytocin release, and the symptoms recede once oxytocin decreases (Uvnäs Moberg, 2015). Prolactin, the other principal hormone in lactation, is released more gradually, 10 to 20 minutes after the onset of breastfeeding, so it is unlikely to be involved in the symptoms.

Oxytocin, a hormone associated with well-being and calm, has another function: It helps mothers protect their babies and can trigger aggression and is linked to negative feelings in the mother,

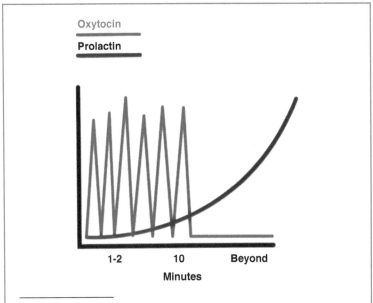

The release of oxytocin vs. prolactin during suckling. During the first 10 minutes of having your baby at the breast, oxytocin is released in pulses. Prolactin does not start to rise until about 10 minutes after the onset of suckling (Kendall-Tackett & Uvnas-Moberg, 2018).

such as fear and anger when she senses threat to her baby. This reaction is activated when the mother perceives the environment as hostile or dangerous (Uvnäs Moberg, 2015).

With this in mind, we hypothesized that the symptoms of D-MER resemble a short-term expression of maternal aggression, that the aggression side of oxytocin was being triggered instead of the love and bonding side.

Symptoms of D-MER do not mean that mothers have negative feelings toward their babies. Rather, we believe that the burst of oxytocin activates, by mistake, mothers' defense reactions rather than the more positive feelings normally associated with breastfeeding (Uvnäs Moberg, 2015).

What Will Help?

As so little is known about D-MER, we used hormonal research to suggest some things that might help (Uvnäs Moberg & Kendall-Tackett, 2018). Milk ejection has become paired with the stress response. The goal is to rewire oxytocin so that it is no longer triggering the fight-or-flight response via classical conditioning. A similar process is involved in PTSD: normal sensations become paired with a fear response. Using the literature from PTSD, we hypothesized that it is possible to re-pair milk ejection with positive sensations and unpair it from the stress response.

Promote Safety

With D-MER, breastfeeding triggers the fight-or-flight response, which suggests that mothers do not feel safe. The primary strategy, then, is to help mothers with D-MER feel safe. In the early days, mothers need to be surrounded by people they trust.

Skin-to-Skin Contact and Massage

Birth is extremely stressful for both mother and baby. Skin-to-skin contact has a powerful antistress effect and can help counter the feelings associated with D-MER (Bystrova et al., 2003). Oxytocin receptors in the skin release more oxytocin and have stronger links to the antistress system than suckling and milk ejection (Uvnäs Moberg, 2015). By triggering a stronger response, skin contact could counter the negative effect associated with milk ejection and possibly help re-pair milk ejection with positive sensations.

Warmth

Cold activates the stress system, which can intensify D-MER symptoms. To counter that reaction, warmth can help. A hot pack around the neck, a blanket, or possibly a warm foot soak, can warm mothers and release oxytocin, which may counter the negative association of oxytocin and let-down.

Mindfulness

Mindfulness is a technique that involves paying attention to breathing and observing but not engaging with thoughts (Sanford, 2018, 2019). Mindfulness might also be helpful when mothers are flooded with the negative thoughts associated with D-MER. With mindfulness, mothers focus on their breathing, are in the present moment, and treat themselves with compassion. Negative thoughts they are experiencing are *thoughts*, not *facts*. Patient education about the symptoms can also help, so mothers know these symptoms will go away soon. Instead, when these feelings strike, you can tell yourself, "These symptoms will stop in a few minutes," "These feelings don't mean I'm a bad mom," or "I will concentrate on my breathing until I feel better."

Dr. Diane Sanford's (2019) book about mindfulness for postpartum women is also helpful.

This mother described how changing her thinking about her symptoms made it easier for her to cope:

> Before I knew what it was, it was very disconcerting and not the feelings I expected to have while breastfeeding. When I understood what was happening, then I could manage through those few minutes by distracting myself and positive self-talk, like reassuring myself that it wasn't really me, it would go away soon, and I would feel better. (Uvnäs Moberg & Kendall-Tackett, 2018, p. 28)

A key way to cope with D-MER is to not ruminate on these negative feelings, wondering what they mean and what they say about you as a mother. If you think about them, and chew on them, and feel ashamed of them, your thoughts can compound the negative effects. Try to picture these negative thoughts as birds flying over your head. Let them go. To paraphrase from Martin Luther, you can't stop birds from flying overhead, but you do not need to allow them to nest in your hair.

Control Insulin

In *The Breastfeeding Atlas*, Barbara Wilson-Clay shared a case study of a mother with D-MER. She told the mother to eat 4 ounces of protein at each meal to maintain her blood sugar levels (Wilson-Clay & Hoover, 2017). The mother noted the following:

> Adding protein helped my symptoms dramatically!!! I wonder if my blood sugars were just fluctuating like crazy. I was carb loading just to try to keep something in my stomach to control my nausea. (p. 141)

This case is of interest because suckling and oxytocin release insulin (Uvnäs Moberg, 2015). When insulin levels are too high, adding protein and removing excessive amounts of carbohydrates from the diet can moderate insulin levels, which may be contributing to symptoms.

BREASTFEEDING AND MENTAL HEALTH

Breastfeeding lowers mothers' risk of mental health conditions, but mothers can still develop postpartum depression, anxiety, and PTSD. D-MER is not a postpartum mental disorder per se, but it can be distressing for mothers. The next two chapters provide more detailed information about trauma, which many mothers have experienced. Traumatic experiences include birth trauma, a history of childhood abuse or adversity, violence, and sexual assault.

CHAPTER 15

BREASTFEEDING AFTER A TRAUMATIC BIRTH EXPERIENCE

A difficult or traumatic birth can upend your life and change the way you see the world. As with other types of trauma, a difficult or traumatic birth can happen suddenly and without warning. You disconnect from others, including your partner and your baby. You blame others and yourself. You keep replaying the events of your birth over and over. Some mothers worry that they are losing their minds. If you feel this way, take heart; these are normal reactions following a traumatic event. It possibly could be posttraumatic stress disorder (PTSD).

PTSD is something we think of when we talk about combat, natural disaster, or sexual assault—not birth. I first noticed the connection between birth experiences and PTSD when interviewing women for a book on postpartum depression in 1992. At that time, you couldn't officially diagnose a woman who experienced a traumatic birth with PTSD because the event you experienced had to be "outside the range of normal human experience." Birth obviously didn't fit. Fortunately, the diagnostic criteria have changed, and it's now possible to diagnose childbirth-related PTSD. The new criteria in the *Diagnostic and Statistical Manual of Mental Disorders* (fifth ed.; American Psychiatric Association, 2013) describe traumatic events as death or threatened death, actual or threatened serious injury, or actual or threatened sexual violation. Birth can contain elements of all three. Even if you don't meet full criteria for PTSD, you can still have symptoms that can interfere with your life.

PERCENTAGE OF WOMEN WHO EXPERIENCE TRAUMATIC BIRTH

Traumatic births are common in many parts of the world, including the United States. Childbirth Connections' Listening to Mothers' Survey II included a nationally representative sample of 1,573 mothers in the United States. Nine percent of these mothers met full criteria for childbirth-related PTSD, and 18% had posttraumatic symptoms (PTS; Beck et al., 2011). This percentage may seem low, so let me give you a number to compare it with. The percentage of people in lower Manhattan who met the full criteria for PTSD after 9/11 was 7.5% (Galea et al., 2003). In Beck et al.'s (2011) study, the percentage of women who met full criteria for PTSD following childbirth was *higher* than it was after a major terrorist attack.

Birth trauma also happens outside the United States. A study from Australia found a lower rate of full-criterion PTSD—6.3% at 12 weeks—but 46% of those mothers described their births as traumatic (Alcorn et al., 2010). Most of the women in this study did not develop PTSD, but were still affected. The rates of postpartum depression and anxiety were higher than the percentage who reported their births as traumatic, demonstrating that traumatic birth was not the only cause, but certainly contributed: Depression ranged from 47% to 66% at 4 to 6 weeks; anxiety ranged from 58% to 74%.

It doesn't have to be this way. The model of care makes a difference. What if women gave birth in countries with a midwifery (vs. obstetric) model of care, where women have continuous labor support, birth is treated as a normal physiologic event, and rates of interventions are low? In one such country, Sweden, out of 1,224 mothers, 1.3% had PTSD, and 9% described their births as traumatic (Söderquist et al., 2009).

In the Netherlands, where there is a similar model of care, only 15% to 17% of women have cesareans (compared with 32% in the United States), and 9% to 10% have instrumental deliveries. (In the United States, the rate for instrumental deliveries is much lower; 0.5% for forceps and 2.6% for vacuum extraction. One possible explanation is that instrumental deliveries are used more in places like the Netherlands to avoid cesareans.) A study of 907 women from the Netherlands found that 1.2% had PTSD and 9% identified their births as traumatic (Stramrood et al., 2011).

Conversely, there are higher rates of PTSD in countries where the status of women is low. In a study of 400 women in Iran, more than half reported traumatic births at 6 to 8 weeks postpartum, and 20% met full criteria for PTSD (Modarres et al., 2012).

WHAT MAKES AN EXPERIENCE NEGATIVE?

Some births seem awful to outsiders, yet mothers feel positively about them. Other women have births that seem "perfect" on paper, yet the mothers are deeply troubled. What makes the difference? A recent review of 21 studies found that the strongest predictor of birth trauma was neither emergencies nor the personality of the mother; it was the quality of the provider interaction (Simpson & Catling, 2016). If the provider was cold, harsh, or critical during labor, mothers were more likely to consider the birth traumatic. These findings support the earlier results from Beck (2004), who found that women's perceived level of care was an important factor. If women felt cared for during their births, they were more likely to perceive them positively. In contrast, if women described their care providers as cold, mechanical, or uncaring or that they felt degraded or raped after their experiences, they were more likely to have birth trauma.

Another factor was women's sense of power and control. Women who felt like they had no control were more likely to react negatively. Perceived control also explains why women can feel positively about an objectively difficult birth: If they felt that they had a say in what happened to them versus others making the decisions about their care (Kendall-Tackett, 2010a, 2014). Beck (2004) also noted that women trusted the hospital staff to provide safe care—trusting not only their lives but also the lives of their babies. If the doctors and nurses provided unsafe care, women were more likely to have birth trauma. In summarizing these women's experiences, Beck noted the following:

> Women who perceived that they had experienced traumatic births viewed the site of their labor and delivery as a battlefield. While engaged in battle, their protective layers were stripped away, leaving them exposed to the onslaught of birth trauma. Stripped from these women were their individuality, dignity, control, communication, caring, trust, and support and reassurance. (p. 34)

In a meta-ethnography of 10 qualitative studies on birth trauma, women indicated that they felt traumatized by their care providers and experienced care as dehumanizing, disrespectful, and uncaring (Elmir et al., 2010). The women had worse symptoms if they felt invisible and out of control, and they also used words like *barbaric, intrusive, horrific, inhumane,* and *degrading.* Their experiences were worse if large numbers of people watched their births without their consent. The mothers described feeling out of control, powerless, and vulnerable. They felt that they were unable to make informed decisions about their care and felt coerced into procedures just to make it stop.

In the book *Battling Over Birth* (Oparah et al., 2018), the authors described the results of a mixed-method study of Black women in California. The authors were interested in the large disparity in maternal mortality between Black and White women; Black women were 4 times more likely to die than their White counterparts. Black women described several difficulties they encountered, including refusal to listen to women's wisdom about their bodies; not respecting women's boundaries or bodily autonomy; stereotyping based on race, class, age, or marital status; and suppressing advocacy and self-advocacy.

WOMEN'S PERCEPTION OF EVENTS

A recent study from Denmark ($N = 1,480$) found that women's perception of events during their births was an important predictor of birth trauma (Garthus-Niegel et al., 2018). Dr. Charles Figley (1986), in his seminal book *Trauma and Its Wake: Vol. 2,* provided an excellent framework for understanding what makes an experience traumatic. He noted that an event would be troubling to the extent that it is *sudden, overwhelming*, and *dangerous*. Thinking about this framework and the events of your birth, was it

Sudden: Did your birth quickly change from "fine" to dangerous? Did anyone take the time to explain what was happening to you?

Overwhelming: Did you feel swept away by the hospital routine or disconnected from what was happening? Did you have general anesthesia? Was your baby taken away?

Dangerous: Was your delivery a medical emergency? Did you develop a life-threatening complication? Did you think you or your baby would die?

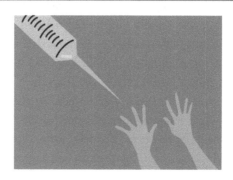

Birth interventions can lead to trauma symptoms if they are sudden, dangerous, and overwhelming.

IMPACT OF TRAUMATIC BIRTH ON BREASTFEEDING

Your birth can influence your early breastfeeding experience. Beck and Watson's (2008) and Beck's (2011) qualitative studies demonstrated that women had mixed feelings about breastfeeding after a traumatic birth. For some women, breastfeeding was unpleasant and reminded them of their births. For others, breastfeeding was healing. Here is what some of them said:

> The flashbacks to the birth was terrible. I wanted to forget about it and the pain, so stopping breastfeeding would get me a bit closer to my "normal" self again. (Beck, 2011, p. 306)

Another mother had a flashback while her baby was on her chest. I suspect that the providers had no idea this was happening with this mother. They were thinking, "skin-to-skin is good," but skin-to-skin reminded the mother of when she thought her baby had died:

> I had flashbacks to the birth every time I would feed him. When he was put on me in the hospital, he wasn't breathing, and he

was blue. I kept picturing this; and could still feel what it was like. Breastfeeding him was a similar position as to the way he was put on me. (Beck & Watson, p. 234)

In the next story, we see why it's so important to address birth trauma promptly. The most important goal following a traumatic birth is for you to connect with your baby.

> The first 5 months of my baby's life (before I got help) are a virtual blank. I dutifully nursed him every 2–3 hours on demand, but I rarely made eye contact with him and dumped him in his crib as soon as I was done. I thought that if it were not for breast-feeding, I could go the whole day without interacting with him at all. (Beck & Watson, 2008, p. 235)

In contrast, some mothers not only were able to breastfeed, but they found it to be tremendously healing. For example, one mother said this:

> Breastfeeding was a timeout from the pain in my head. It was a "current reality"—a way to cling onto some "real life," whereas all the trauma that continued to live on in my head belonged to the past, even though I couldn't seem to keep it there. (Beck & Watson, p. 233)

Her story makes sense from a physiological point of view. Breast-feeding temporarily turned off the stress response, which allowed her a break from the continuous loop that was playing in her head. Another mother felt that breastfeeding was important for her self-esteem as a mother:

> Breastfeeding became my focus for overcoming the birth and proving to everyone else and mostly myself that there was something that I could do right. It was part of my crusade, so to speak, to prove myself as a mother. (Beck & Watson, 2008, p. 233)

This mother shared how breastfeeding gave her confidence in her body. She viewed herself as a failure following her birth, and breastfeeding gave her a chance to do something positive:

> My body's ability to produce milk, and so the sustenance to keep my baby alive also helped to restore my faith in my body, which at some core level, I felt had really let me down, due to a terrible pregnancy, labor, and birth. It helped build my confidence in my body and as a mother. It helped me heal and feel connected to my baby. (Beck & Watson, p. 233)

BIRTH INTERVENTIONS INFLUENCE BREASTFEEDING AND DEPRESSIVE SYMPTOMS

A stressful birth influences breastfeeding because it activates the stress system, which suppresses oxytocin. High cortisol levels suppress prolactin, the hormone involved in milk production. The most immediate effect of traumatic birth is on lactogenesis II, which can cause early problems for the baby such as jaundice and weight loss. Other birth interventions can also cause downstream breastfeeding problems. A study of 5,332 mothers in the United Kingdom found that women had more breastfeeding problems at 3 months postpartum if they had forceps-assisted and unplanned cesarean births (Rowlands & Redshaw, 2012). Again, it's likely that stress made initial breastfeeding difficult, and the effect reverberated 3 months later.

Our data with 6,410 new mothers were also quite interesting (Kendall-Tackett et al., 2015). We found that 83% of mothers who had unassisted vaginal deliveries were exclusively breastfeeding. If mothers had any other type of birth, their rate of exclusive breastfeeding ranged from 69% to 71%, a highly significant difference. Although the mother's perceptions of her birth can influence her vulnerability to depression or PTSD, there may be a more fundamental physiology that is influencing her breastfeeding experience. Birth interventions can influence oxytocin and prolactin, the two hormones necessary for breastfeeding, which can make it more difficult to establish breastfeeding in the early days (Grajeda & Pérez-Escamilla, 2002; Uvnäs Moberg et al., 2020). That can influence whether breastfeeding is exclusive.

Our data on birth interventions and depressive symptoms were also interesting and, in some ways, unexpected. When I first looked at these data, I fully expected that women who had emergency cesareans would have higher depressive symptoms. We were surprised to find that women who had planned cesareans had even higher rates. In contrast, women who had unplanned (nonemergency) cesareans had low rates. When I tried to think about why women who had unplanned cesareans had such low rates, I thought of two mothers I knew who both tried for a vaginal birth after cesarean but ended up with second cesareans. Although it was not what they wanted, they were both happy with their births. Everyone was calm; it wasn't an emergency; they had good support and felt that their wishes were respected.

The high depressive symptoms in women who had planned cesareans was another puzzle. In talking with oxytocin expert Dr. Kerstin Uvnäs Moberg, we believe that these findings may be due to no trial of labor. During labor, every time the baby's head presses against the cervix, there is a release of oxytocin (Uvnäs Moberg, 2015). Women who do not go through labor do not have these surges of oxytocin, which means lower levels postpartum. Lower oxytocin means more activation of the stress system, with increases the risk for depression (Kendall-Tackett, 2017).

Epidurals are a common birth intervention that can influence both breastfeeding and mental health. This doesn't mean that mothers should never have them because they are sometimes medically necessary. Instead, I would like to see providers acknowledge that they can have downstream effects (Kendall-Tackett et al., 2015). In our study, we found that epidurals were related to higher depressive symptoms, even after we controlled for all the other risk factors for depression, and only 42% of mothers who had epidurals were exclusively breastfeeding. If you had one, you can still breastfeed, but there may be challenges (discussed later in the chapter).

WHAT YOU CAN DO

If you have had a negative birth experience, you cannot change that. There are, however, a number of steps that you can take to make peace with your experience. Here are some things that other mothers have found useful. Keep in mind that coming to terms with a negative birth experience is a process that can take months. Don't be discouraged if it doesn't happen overnight or if you seem to have bad days. You can overcome this!

Some Possible Challenges With Breastfeeding

Although not always true, a difficult birth can lead to some breastfeeding challenges. I want to be realistic but also encouraging. Knowledge is power. There can be problems, but with good support, you can meet your breastfeeding goals.

Delay in Lactogenesis II

One of the immediate issues following a traumatic birth is delayed lactogenesis II. For most women, lactogenesis II happens around Days 3 to 4. Following a stressful birth, it can be Day 5, 6, or longer. If you've had a stressful birth, you may try to counter the effects by increasing the times you empty your breasts, either by baby or using a pump. Aim for a minimum of 10 times a day, using breast massage and compressions as you nurse, or use a pump until your milk becomes more abundant (Walker, 2018). I've listed more strategies in Chapter 8. If you have any concerns, have your health care provider or lactation specialist monitor the situation and check your baby's weight.

Doing any amount of supplementation can feel so discouraging, and you may be tempted to give it up. What I would encourage you to do instead is to remind yourself that this situation is a temporary bump in the road. Ask your partner or support person to be with you on this too. The goal of brief supplementation, preferably at the breast, is to get breastfeeding back on track. Being able to meet your breastfeeding goals will also support your mental health.

You can reevaluate your plan in a week. Within a week, lactogenesis II will have occurred and you can realistically evaluate what you want to do from there. Ideally, all will be well. If there is another challenge to tackle, I'd encourage you to address one bit at a time. Overwise, it can feel impossible. It's not, but be sure to be extra kind to yourself.

PAIN

Pain can also be a potent trigger for trauma symptoms. If you are experiencing pain, be sure to see a provider who addresses it. If you are told to "keep doing what you're doing," go see someone else. It's vital for your mental health that pain is addressed. Please don't try to tough it out.

SKIN-TO-SKIN CONTACT

After a difficult birth, skin-to-skin contact may feel too intense. If it does, you can limit how much you have. The most important bit is your baby's cheek on your breast. Everything else is optional. On

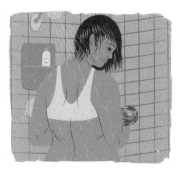

Some mothers find that bathing with their baby is a great way to reconnect after a difficult birth.

the other hand, skin-to-skin might help you feel better. The amount that you have is up to you. Experiment and do as much or as little as you are comfortable with. Some mothers enjoy sharing a bath or shower with their babies and find it's a great way to reconnect or even "rebirth" their babies. You might give that a try to see if it helps.

Process Your Experience

Find a person who will not try to minimize your feelings or give you a pep talk. You might also find it useful to contact one of the support organizations that can validate your feelings and help you come to terms with what happened. Some women have found that going to a therapist helps. Another option is to write about your experience. If you'd like to give that a try, the book *Writing to Heal* (Pennebaker, 2004) will help you get the most out of this activity. Writing gives you a chance to express your feelings without fear of censure.

Learn as Much as You Can About Your Experience

Consider getting copies of your medical records. You have a right to see them, and they may help you understand what happened. If you feel comfortable, talk with your health care provider or someone else who can help you understand what happened during your birth. It also helps to read books that might put your birth experience in a broader perspective. You might particularly enjoy Dr. Christine Morton's (Morton & Clift, 2014) epic book *Birth Ambassadors: Doulas and the Re-Emergence of Women-Supported Birth in America.* This type of reading will do much to validate your experience and help you understand it. You may be angry (or you may get angry for the first time), but eventually, the experience will not dominate your thoughts. If you plan to have another baby, the information will make you an informed consumer. If you are considering another pregnancy, you might want to hire a doula, get a different provider, or change hospitals. You might also consider a birth center or home birth.

Your Partner May Have Also Been Traumatized

A traumatic birth can cause problems between you and your partner. Your partner may have also felt powerless and swept away by the experience. This may be especially difficult for men, who feel that it is their job to protect—and that can be almost impossible in a hospital, where your partner is almost as powerless as you. He might feel as though he failed to protect you and might react to his negative feelings by being angry with you. Same-sex partners may experience similar difficulties in the hospital setting but may also encounter prejudice and homophobia from hospital staff. If your partner is also traumatized, they might not be effective emotional support for you. This can also cause problems between you. In this

251

case, be honest about your feelings and try to find outside support together. If your partner is unwilling to work with you to resolve your birth experience, I'd encourage you to seek help alone.

Birth Is Only the Beginning of a Lifelong Relationship With Your Baby

You may feel bad that you "allowed" this to happen, which can compound your already shaky confidence as a mother. First of all, you are not responsible for what happened to you. Second, this doesn't have to govern what happens next. Recognize that motherhood is a role you gradually grow into. The difficult beginning you had is not the blueprint for the rest of your mothering career. A negative birth experience can affect your relationship with your baby, but it does not have to. This is why it is vital for you to get the support you need as soon as possible.

Forgive Yourself

Many women feel that they have somehow failed. They blame themselves for what happened and played the "if only" game: "If only I had been stronger . . ." "If only I had checked out the doctor/hospital more carefully . . ." "If only I had gone to a different prenatal class . . ." The "if only's" are endless. Recognize that you did the best you could under the circumstances and with the knowledge you had at the time, and let yourself off the hook!

CONCLUSION

Take good care of yourself and actively search for support. You may face some breastfeeding difficulties and challenges to your emotional state. The early days can be rough. However, many mothers have overcome difficult beginnings, and I am confident that you can too.

CHAPTER 16

BREASTFEEDING AFTER CHILDHOOD ABUSE, ADVERSITIES, AND SEXUAL ASSAULT

Childhood trauma, sexual assault, and partner violence are surprisingly common among childbearing women. When mothers have histories of abuse, they often wonder if breastfeeding is even possible for them. You may be surprised to learn that it's not only possible, but it can lessen your trauma symptoms. Before I show you those studies, I want to provide a brief overview of what we know about the impact of violence against women and how it influences their parenting and breastfeeding experiences. I'll share stories from the many women I've spoken with. They have been my best teachers.

ADVERSE CHILDHOOD EXPERIENCES

The term *adverse childhood experiences* (or ACEs) came from a large study in the late 1990s of 17,000 patients at the Kaiser Permanente Hospital in San Diego (Felitti et al., 1998). The researchers, Drs. Vincent Felitti and Robert Anda, recognized that to understand the effects of abuse, you needed to include all the types of abuse and adversity a person had experienced during childhood. In their study, the more types of ACEs a person had experienced, the higher their risk for serious health problems as adults. ACEs fall into four main categories. Each one of the types within the four categories counts for one ACE.

Child Maltreatment

This category includes all types of childhood abuse (physical, sexual, and emotional) and physical and emotional neglect.

Parental Impairment

Parents can be impaired as caregivers by using substances, having a mental illness (including depression), and being involved in criminal activity. This category also includes parental partner violence. Children who observe partner violence show signs of abuse, even if they've never been abused themselves.

Parental Loss

Loss of a parent through death or divorce has a significant effect. Especially as you transition into new motherhood, the loss of a parent, particularly your own mother, can be particularly difficult.

Factors Associated With Lower Socioeconomic Status

In recent years, researchers have added another layer to the original ACE study. They have noted that things that happen in a family take place in the context of a community. If the family is healthy, those relationships buffer the negative effects of poverty. However, if the family is vulnerable, lower socioeconomic status can compound the negative effects. These factors include community violence, unsafe housing, food insecurity, and lack of access to medical care.

How Common Are ACEs, Violence, and Sexual Assault?

ACEs and sexual assault are remarkably common. For example, one study from the Boston area compared 3,500 mothers in two

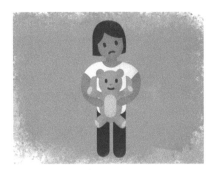

Childhood adversities are remarkably common. The more types of adversities a child experiences, the higher their risk for adult health problems and perinatal mood disorders.

neighborhoods, one in the inner city and the other an affluent suburb. They found that the rate of lifetime abuse was remarkably similar: 46% in the suburbs and 57% in the inner city (Rich-Edwards et al., 2011).

From our sample of 6,410 mothers, we found that 16% had been raped, 25% reported contact child sexual abuse, 32% reported that their parents abused substances, 34% reported physical abuse, and 36% reported that one or both of their parents were depressed (Kendall-Tackett et al., 2013). Although the mothers in our study had a wide range of incomes, by education level, our sample was predominantly middle class: 73% had a bachelor's degree or higher.

DO ACEs OR SEXUAL ASSAULT INFLUENCE BREASTFEEDING?

Several recent studies examined the effects of childhood abuse, sexual assault, and partner violence on breastfeeding. Two of the earliest studies surprised people. One found a significantly higher intention to breastfeed (Benedict et al., 1994) and the other found higher breastfeeding initiation (Prentice et al., 2002) among women who had been sexually abused. Those findings seemed counterintuitive. People assumed that abuse survivors, particularly sexual abuse survivors, would never want to breastfeed. A more recent study by Coles et al. (2016) found that women with a history of child sexual abuse breastfed at similar rates to nonabused women. However, a study from Canada found similar rates of breastfeeding initiation between ACE survivors and nonabused women, but ACE survivors were less likely to exclusively breastfeed (Ukah et al., 2016).

A study from Norway found that women with a history of childhood abuse were more likely to stop breastfeeding before 4 months (Sørbø et al., 2015). Women were 41% more likely to stop if they had experienced one or more types of violence, 40% more likely if they had experienced violence in the last 12 months, 28% more likely if the perpetrator was known to them, and 22% more likely if they experienced childhood sexual abuse. This study included more than 50,000 participants.

These findings show that abuse survivors start breastfeeding at the same rates as nonabused women, but they tend to stop earlier. This tells me that we need to continue supporting these mothers beyond the immediate postpartum period.

BREASTFEEDING CAN HELP YOU OVERCOME THE EFFECTS OF ABUSE

Researchers have found that breastfeeding is particularly helpful for abuse survivors. The first major finding was that breastfeeding stops the cycle of abuse. Breastfeeding is a powerful physiological mechanism that downregulates *your* stress system. It's part of nature's brilliant design that recognizes that even if you had abusive, neglectful, or absent parents, your body gives you a chance to do things differently.

Dr. Lane Strathearn and his colleagues (2009) found that breastfeeding lowered the risk of child abuse and neglect. Their sample included 7,223 mother–infant pairs, and they followed them for 15 years. During that time, there were 500 documented (by Child Protection) cases where mothers either abused or neglected their children. If mothers breastfed for at least 4 months, they were 3.8 times less likely to neglect their children and 2.6 times less likely to physically abuse them. Strathearn and colleagues attributed some of this effect to increased oxytocin leading to increased mother–infant bonding.

Keep their findings in mind when you review our data (Kendall-Tackett et al., 2013). When we looked at sleep and maternal well-being, we had already found that exclusive breastfeeding differed physiologically from both mixed-feeding and exclusive formula-feeding, and there was no difference between mixed- and formula-feeding for these variables (Kendall-Tackett et al., 2011). Eventually, we combined mixed- and formula-feeding groups and analyzed our data by exclusive versus nonexclusive breastfeeding (EBF vs. non-EBF).

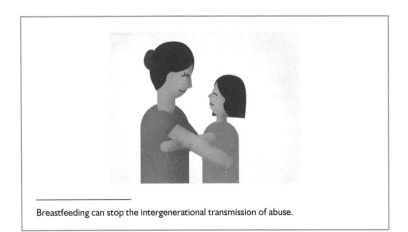

Breastfeeding can stop the intergenerational transmission of abuse.

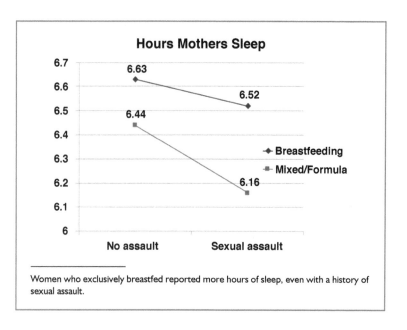

Women who exclusively breastfed reported more hours of sleep, even with a history of sexual assault.

In our sample, there were 994 women who reported that they had been raped. Across the board, these women had lower measures of well-being, sleep, and mental health than the women in the sample who had not been raped (Kendall-Tackett et al., 2013). On the basis of previous studies, this was expected. We also found that women who had been raped exclusively breastfed at exactly the same rate as their nonassaulted counterparts (78% for each group).

In the next set of analyses, we combined data on sexual assault status with exclusive versus nonexclusive breastfeeding and were stunned at the results. We first looked at number of hours that mothers slept. EBF women slept longer overall, even if they had been assaulted. The amount of sleep was significantly lower in the non-EBF women.

Minutes to get to sleep had a similar pattern. Minutes to get to sleep and total sleep hours are the two strongest sleep-related

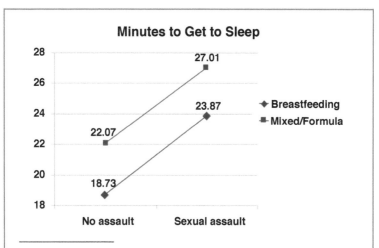

Minutes to Get to Sleep

Minutes to get to sleep is another key predictor of postpartum depression. Although the number is higher if women have a history of sexual assault, it is significantly lower than for nonexclusively breastfeeding mothers.

predictors of postpartum depression (Dørheim et al., 2009b). Among mothers with a history of sexual assault, exclusively breastfeeding mothers took fewer minutes to get to sleep than their non-EBF counterparts.

With both of these variables, there is an elevated risk of depression in all mothers with a history of assault, so these mothers will need support even if they are exclusively breastfeeding. However, the exclusively breastfeeding mothers are at significantly lower risk.

We also found that mothers who exclusively breastfed had significantly fewer depressive symptoms, but they were still elevated for all mothers with a history of sexual assault.

My favorite data were on the effect of exclusive breastfeeding on mothers' anger and irritability. The EBF mothers were equal to the nonassaulted mothers. In contrast, there was a spike of anger and irritability in the non-EBF mothers. The pattern is characteristic of

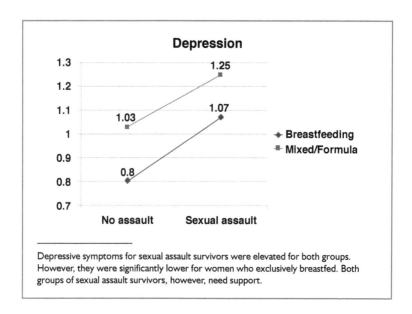

Depression

Depressive symptoms for sexual assault survivors were elevated for both groups. However, they were significantly lower for women who exclusively breastfed. Both groups of sexual assault survivors, however, need support.

PTSD and reflects a hypersensitive stress response (Kiecolt-Glaser et al., 2007). In our article, we hypothesized that breastfeeding downregulated the stress response, providing at least a partial respite from trauma symptoms (Kendall-Tackett et al., 2013). Although EBF doesn't completely eliminate trauma's effects, it lessens them, which may be enough to help you cope with the stresses of new motherhood.

Thinking back to the Strathearn et al. (2009) study, they found that mothers were less likely to abuse or neglect their children if they breastfed for at least 4 months. Can breastfeeding prevent child abuse and help you parent differently? Yes! Here's the physiology of it: If you're less prone to be angry and irritable, you're going to be less likely to snap at your kids and respond abusively.

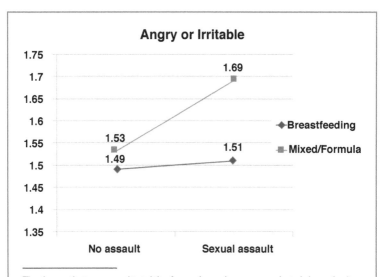

The sharp spike in anger and irritability for mothers who are not exclusively breastfeeding is characteristic of posttraumatic stress disorder. The most striking finding of this study was the low level of anger and irritability in exclusively breastfeeding mothers. It demonstrates that breastfeeding downregulated the stress response.

You might also wonder whether breastfeeding continues to help you even after you've stopped. Two studies suggest that it does. The first is the Strathearn et al. (2009) study, which was conducted over 15 years. Breastfeeding at least 4 months lowered the risk of child maltreatment over the entire 15-year study period. The second study is a 14-year longitudinal study that looked at children's mental health, which presumably would be affected by child maltreatment. In this study, if babies were breastfed for at least 12 months, children's mental health was better at every time point up to age 14 (Oddy et al., 2010). One explanation is that responsive parenting led to a secure attachment (breastfeeding does not work unless babies are responded to). Another intriguing possibility is that the constant upregulation of oxytocin during breastfeeding permanently changed the hyperactivity of the stress system. (An overactive stress system is common in abuse survivors. Oxytocin may have brought it down to a more normal level.) Lower anger and irritability may have improved parenting ability.

SOME SPECIFIC ISSUES RELATED TO BREASTFEEDING

Breastfeeding has many benefits for abuse survivors, but you may still encounter some challenges. Although we saw that sexual assault survivors breastfed at the same rate as nonassaulted women, the subjective experience is not always positive. EBF provides the best trauma-reducing effects, but breastfeed as much as you can tolerate. Several years ago, I spoke with one young woman who had been raped by classmates in junior high. She never told anyone what happened—not even her husband. I was the first person she had told. She breastfed four children but said to me that she had "never liked it." I asked her why she was doing it. She said, "It is important. I never liked it, but I learned to tolerate it, and that was enough."

Mothers have told me that their breastfeeding experiences ranged from positive to negative. My approach has always been to do whatever works. If it's exclusive breastfeeding you want, that's what we'll work toward. If it's exclusive pumping, we'll work toward that. (Although exclusive pumping is not always the answer. I worked with one mother for several months, and she told me that the pump was much harder to cope with than her baby at the breast.) From a physiological side, exclusive breastfeeding has advantages for you, but if mixed-feeding is all that you can handle, that's okay. Every bit of your milk your baby gets helps, and you benefit from the close contact with your baby.

SOME ASPECTS OF BREASTFEEDING THAT CAN BE TRIGGERING

Some things in the immediate postpartum period can trigger trauma symptoms. If you start to feel anxious or angry, take a breath and jot down a few notes to see if you can figure out what is happening. There may be a workaround.

Birth

Many aspects of hospital settings can be particularly difficult for trauma survivors, such as lying flat, exposing your private parts to strangers, having people observe your birth without your permission, repeated pelvic exams, physical restraints, and pain. Nurses or lactation consultants who grab your breasts to assist the baby can also trigger you.

Intense Physical Contact

Skin-to-skin contact, although normally a positive thing, can feel overwhelming if you have a hyperactive stress system. Therefore, acknowledge that feeling and take it a bit at a time. Perhaps you can limit contact to only have your baby's cheek on your breast. It's important that you feel okay. Don't grit your way through it. If it's too much, limit the amount.

Pain

Pain can also trigger trauma survivors, which is all the more reason to get some help if it hurts. Your stress system is already primed to respond and overrespond. You don't need to add fuel to the fire. Your comfort is important, and you shouldn't be in pain.

PARENTING CHALLENGES

If you never received good parenting, finding your way in the beginning can be challenging. I've met so many trauma survivors who want to do the right thing and are actively looking for role models. This is when parenting organizations truly shine. They can model parenting practices and how to do things well. However, there are some potential pitfalls, which I would like to help you avoid.

Intense Need to Do Everything Right

If you experienced childhood trauma, you might try hard to be a perfect mother, where even your innermost thoughts are always loving and supportive. It's a nice thought, but it isn't reality. It's okay to occasionally get annoyed with your kids. That doesn't make you a bad mother; it makes you a human being. It's lashing out during those moments of pique that we want to avoid, which will be easier if you recognize that you don't have to be perfect to be a good parent.

It's Okay to Set Boundaries

In my early days as a La Leche League leader, there was a mother in our group who had had some horrific things happen to her in childhood, and her first birth was beyond awful. Her second birth was better, but day-to-day life with an infant and toddler was too much. One day, she came in looking really wrung out and she said, "I never thought my life would be like this. I'm sitting on the couch with my shirt up with a baby on one side and my toddler on the other side." She was trying to do the "right" thing, but it made her miserable. The senior leaders both said to her, "You don't have to do this. You can nurse them one at a time. You can wean your toddler. You don't have to do this." I was impressed. They gave her permission to set some limits, probably for the first time in her life.

The same is true for you. If something is not sitting right with you or makes your skin crawl, step back and see if you can figure out what's bothering you. Is it exposing yourself? Is it too much skin time? Is it feeling trapped in your four walls? If you can figure out what's bothering you, you can work through it. It's okay to do things differently.

SHOULD YOU TELL PEOPLE?

I've been teaching health care providers about this for the past 2 decades, telling them that they don't have a right to information about patients' history of abuse. This means that you don't have to tell people if you don't want to; it's none of their business. Providers sometimes think that if they ask patients, they'll learn the truth. I have found that when patients say "No," it can mean, "I neither know nor trust you" or "no, it didn't happen." A lactation consultant recently told me that she included questions about abuse and assault on her intake form. She saw one mother 10 times, and each time, the mother said "no" when asked about trauma history. On the 11th time, the mother said "yes," saying, "I didn't know you, so I said no."

If you are comfortable with a provider and feel safe, it's perfectly appropriate for you to share your information. Otherwise, if it feels iffy, feel free to withhold it. This is a boundary you can set for yourself.

WHAT YOU CAN DO

Past abuse can influence many areas of your life. Fortunately, there is much you can do to heal. Here are suggestions about where to start.

Process Your Experience

To heal, you'll need a way to process events from your childhood. Professional therapy can help. Be sure to seek out someone you like and have a rapport with. Some of my clients have been in and out of therapy for years. They go back when life gets stressful. Therapy can help you to let go of distorted beliefs you may have about yourself. During childhood, you may have internalized messages about being stupid, lazy, or dirty, and these thoughts could be influencing you today. Much of the harm that comes from past abuse is related to what you have internalized.

Another way to process traumatic events is through writing. James Pennebaker's (2004) research demonstrates that writing can also heal. Many of the men and women in his studies went through experiences that may be similar to yours. Once they wrote about their lives, they were able to put their traumatic pasts behind them and experienced measurable improvements in their psychological and physical health. Pennebaker's (2004) book *Writing to Heal* has many specific suggestions to help you get the most out of this activity.

Get Support

Recovery from traumatic events takes time. Support from others who have gone through similar experiences can also be important. As a trauma survivor, you are at higher risk for depression, anxiety, and posttraumatic stress disorder. If you are having symptoms, don't ignore them. Your parenting experience will be better if you are not also suffering from a postpartum mental illness. One good thing to come out of COVID was the increased availability of telemedicine options. Even if there is no provider in your community who knows about postpartum mood disorders, you can find someone to see you online. Go to Postpartum Support International for a referral (https://www.postpartum.net). I also suggest that you check out the group

Survivor Moms (https://www.survivormoms.org). They have great resources and books for mothers.

Picture Your Capacity for Wellness

Your experience of childhood abuse or sexual assault can be turned into a strength. Many adult survivors have reported that good eventually came from their bad experiences (this is called *posttraumatic growth*). Your past does not have to rule your future. I've known many trauma survivors who have broken the cycle of abuse and created rich, full lives. They are warm and loving parents. Breastfeeding can support you in these parenting goals.

CONCLUSION

I want to close with a story I heard from a WIC peer counselor in Texas. She came up to me at the break during a conference and said, "Oh, what you said was so true." She then recounted her incredible story. She had been raped for the first time at the age of 3. What followed was a series of sexual assaults. Her mother was using substances and seemed unable or unwilling to protect her. This young woman eventually became a prostitute—and then she got pregnant.

For many young women, an unexpected pregnancy would not be positive and would likely end with another generation of abuse. However, someone helped this young woman breastfeed her baby. She told me that it changed everything for her. She got out of the sex trade and went back to school. She eventually trained to become a WIC breastfeeding peer counselor and was working toward her IBCLC [International Board Certified Lactation Consultant]. She told me that breastfeeding changed her life. It was hard to deny the truth of that. The evidence was there to observe. Is she a perfect mother? No. Is she a loving and good mother? Yes! And you can be too.

VII

MOVING BEYOND THE EARLY DAYS

INTRODUCTION: MOVING BEYOND THE EARLY DAYS

Although it may seem impossible to imagine at the beginning, eventually, you'll reach a period of equilibrium with your new little one, and life will move past the immediate postpartum period. This may include employment outside the home. Employment presents unique challenges for the breastfeeding mother. In this section, I describe the accommodations breastfeeding mothers need in the workplace and the mandates in U.S. federal law. I describe the basics of milk storage, child care for breastfeeding babies, and alternative work arrangements.

My final chapter is on what happens when feeding at the breast isn't an option. Almost every place I go, I meet women who have not been able to reach their breastfeeding goals. One mother was in my class for entrepreneurs. She had had two babies with jaundice and breastfed her first baby for a few weeks before she had to stop. When she encountered a similar problem with her second, her husband said, "Just quit." And she did on Day 2. The experience clearly still bothered her. If you find yourself in that position, all is not lost. There are many ways you can connect with your baby. A secure attachment is still attainable, and that is the ultimate goal.

CHAPTER 17

EMPLOYMENT AND THE BREASTFEEDING MOTHER

Most countries in the industrialized world have laws that govern maternity leave and protect mothers when they go back to work. Unfortunately, the United States is the only industrialized country that does not have paid maternity leave, but some companies offer it, and it may happen for federal workers in the near future. Laws protecting nursing mothers in the United States are of particular interest because they protect a group of mothers that you would not see in other countries: mothers needing to return to work sooner than 6 months postpartum. Many lactation consultants believe that the way we treat our new mothers in the United States is barbaric. I agree, but for now, we have to work with the system we have. These laws can protect you when your breastfeeding is still vulnerable. However, as you will see, having a law or policy, and how it is actually implemented, are often two quite different things.

In this chapter, I provide a brief overview of returning to work as a breastfeeding mother. I also recognize that some women opt to stay home or have a different type of work arrangement. I briefly discuss those options as well. COVID has made many see work differently and realize that many jobs can be done in a variety of ways. As I've had to be necessarily brief in this chapter, I'd like to steer you toward other good sources of information that provide more detail. The KellyMom.com site is a treasure trove, as are *The Business Case for Breastfeeding* (U.S. Office of Women's Health, 2018), the Carolina Global Breastfeeding Institute, and the U.S. Office for Women's Health.

BREASTFEEDING, WORKING, AND U.S. FEDERAL LAW

If you are a breastfeeding mother in the United States, federal law mandates workplace accommodations to protect breastfeeding mothers. This law was part of the Affordable Care Act, which amends the Fair Labor Standards Act (Martin, 2011; U.S. Department of Labor, n.d.). Here are a couple of key provisions:

> Federal law requires employers to provide *reasonable break time* for an employee to express breast milk for her nursing child for one year after the child's birth each time such employee has need to express the milk.

> Employers are also *required to provide a place, other than a bathroom,* that is shielded from view and free from intrusion from coworkers and the public, which may be used by an employee to express breast milk.

> An employer shall not be required to compensate an employee receiving reasonable break time under paragraph 1 for any work time spent for such purpose.

And the gigantic loophole:

> *An employer that employs less than 50 employees shall not be subject to the requirements of this subsection,* if such requirements would impose an undue hardship by causing the employer significant difficulty or expense when considered in relation to the size, financial resources, nature, or structure of the employer's business. (Martin, 2011; U.S. Department of Labor, n.d., emphasis added)

The law doesn't prescribe the number of pumping breaks beyond a "reasonable" number, but the typical is two to three times a day for the first year (Martin, 2011).

PLANNING YOUR LEAVE AND RETURN

Ideally, it's best to have this conversation before you go on leave. If you didn't, you may want to chat with your boss (or human resources department) before you come back.

Talk to Your Employer Before You Go

Planning ahead will ease return. You might feel embarrassed to talk with your boss about breastfeeding, but if you prepare ahead of time and are specific about what you need, it may not be as bad as you expect. Unfortunately, not everyone is nice about it. The point is that you are protected by law and are not asking for favors. Explain that you need time to pump and private space that is not a bathroom and let them know when you plan to return to work. You will feel more comfortable having this talk if you know your rights and the advantages for your employer if you continue breastfeeding (Needels, 2019). It is good for both of you.

What Your Employer Gets

The *Business Case for Breastfeeding* (U.S. Office of Women's Health, 2018) highlights the major employer benefits. You can download this document for your employer.

- *More satisfied and loyal employees.* Training new employees is expensive. By accommodating breastfeeding, they are more likely to retain employees who will be more motivated in their work.

- *Reduced sick time for both moms and their partners for children's illnesses.* Breastfed babies get sick less often because of the immunity passed along through breastmilk.
- *Lower health care costs.* Mothers and babies are less likely to get sick, and thus the costs for insurance are lower (U.S. Office of Women's Health, 2018, n.d.). For two corporations in Southern California, breastfeeding employees had half as many absences related to infant illness as their formula-feeding counterparts. Aetna saved $1,435 per breastfed baby per year. CIGNA saved $240,000 per year in health care costs and another $60,000 per year related to absenteeism (California Breastfeeding Coalition, n.d.).

MATERNITY LEAVE

Returning to work will be easier if you've had at least 3 months of maternity leave. For some mothers, that amount is not possible. A maternity leave of fewer than 3 months is still doable, but it makes sustaining breastfeeding more difficult. Unfortunately, short leaves are common. In the United States, 25% of new mothers return to work by an appalling 2 weeks postpartum. Sustaining breastfeeding will be difficult for these mothers (Lukas, 2019).

Return Gradually

The Office of Women's Health recommends that you plan to come back to work on a Thursday or Friday, which will be a shorter week for you and your baby. Prep your baby by introducing a bottle at least 1 week before you plan to go back to work (Needels, 2019). As many mothers have found, someone else may need to give your baby a bottle because they won't take it from you. Try a couple of different bottles to see which ones your baby prefers.

Get a Quality Breast Pump

You will want a double-electric pump to shorten your time expressing and to help maintain your supply. I'd also recommend a hands-free setup so you can do something else while pumping. Many mothers make their own hands-free setups by cutting holes in a running bra. Your insurance may help cover your pump and accessories, or you may be able to get one from WIC. As a final option, you could rent a pump for the time when you are expressing milk. The cost will be offset by the amount you would have to spend on formula. Familiarize yourself with your pump at least 4 weeks ahead of time and use that time to stockpile some frozen milk.

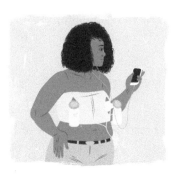

A hands-free setup for your pump allows you to do other things with your hands, like eat your lunch or read a book.

A Sample Daily Schedule

Exclusively breastfeeding mothers need to express milk for 10 to 15 minutes, two or three times per day, and may need more time to get to the place where they can pump (U.S. Office of Women's Health, 2018). Pumping this frequently will help maintain your supply and also provide enough milk for your provider to feed your baby while you are away. Bring your lunch or snacks so you can pump during your breaks or at lunch (Needels, 2019). The Office of Women's Health (2018) gave a sample schedule for a traditional job:

8:00 a.m. Begin work
9:45–10:00 a.m. Use your break to express milk
12:00 p.m. Use your lunch period to express milk
2:30–2:45 p.m. Use your break to express milk
5:00 p.m. Leave work

Allow time to breastfeed your baby right before you leave for work and breastfeed again once you pick up your baby and before you head home. Those times allow you to empty your breasts (and one less time to pump), reconnect with your baby, and relax before you head home and face the nightly routine of dinner, chores, and older children.

WORKPLACE CHALLENGES TO BREASTFEEDING ACCOMMODATIONS

Accommodations for breastfeeding are part of U.S. federal law, yet mothers still encounter barriers and unhelpful colleagues. Even companies designated "baby-friendly" seem to have a disconnect between the official policies and the way they are implemented. A recent qualitative study described some of these women's experiences of returning to work at companies that had applied for and were designated as "baby-friendly workplaces." This study highlights that there is still work to do with regard to making sure that policies get carried out company wide. Following are some of the challenges mothers reported they had encountered (Cheyney et al., 2019a, 2019b).

Not Clear Who to Ask About Breastfeeding Accommodations

This caused confusion and stress and made it more difficult for mothers in the study to continue to express milk.

No Private Space for Expressing Milk

Although there was supposed to be a designated space, it often had no lock, no chairs or no table to put the pump on, and no place to plug in a pump.

> I had to knock and tell my male colleague [who was also her supervisor] that I needed the space. He said that he thought I would only need it once a day, and I was totally stressed out having to describe to him how pumping for a newborn works. (Cheyney et al., 2019b, p. 115)

> Our designated space was a room that also had the only shower in it. So, my coworkers would work out during lunch, and then want to get in there to take a shower. It was awful. I would be in there trying to pump, and they would be outside beating on the door wanting to get a shower.... I just felt humiliated having to walk out there holding my pump and my milk. (Cheyney et al., 2019b, p. 115)

Colleagues Who Think You Are Asking for or Getting Special Privileges

Many women in the study described intimations that they were getting away with something by taking time to pump, even though this was unpaid time. Colleagues didn't understand why this was necessary and made remarks about it.

This is not a gift, it is a right, but it feels like I am asking for a gift. I am only asking for what they already said they thought I should have ... at least in theory. (Cheyney et al., 2019a, p. 108)

There is just so little flexibility, so the burden falls to the new moms to try to find a way to make it work. That was not at all what I needed in trying to go back to work. (Cheyney et al., 2019a, p. 108)

Colleagues might be bothered by milk stored in the communal refrigerator. Some have even contaminated breast milk, thinking that it is all a big joke. One woman shared that a colleague put alcohol in her baby's milk. Having no place to store breastmilk can be a barrier. In breastfeeding-friendly workplaces, nursing rooms have separate refrigerators.

Providing Onsite Pumps in Inaccessible Places

Some companies do a nice thing when they provide pumps for their employees to use. However, these pumps do not help if they are too far away for someone to practically use, as this mother described:

Having access to a pump means something to me that is more than just hey, there is a pump in the building. It means that the worksite helps rather than hinders the process of getting one, then when you get one, there is space to use it, clean it, and store what comes out of it. Otherwise, what good is it? Just having a pump, I mean. (Cheyney et al., 2019b, p. 116)

STORING YOUR MILK

Lactation expert Kelly Bonyata (2012, 2018a), founder of the KellyMom site, recommends storing milk in 1- to 4-ounce portions. Storing it in smaller portions means that you don't waste it if your baby doesn't finish a larger amount. You can combine milk from different pumping sessions. Write the expression date on the storage bag, and use the date of the first expression (if combining them). Before combining milk from different sessions, cool the new milk first and then add it to the older milk. Breastmilk that has soured smells and tastes bad.

You can thaw frozen milk in the refrigerator. If you need to thaw it more quickly, put it under warm running water. If you've previously frozen it, don't refreeze it, but you can keep it in the refrigerator for up to 24 hours. Don't let it sit out at room temperature.

To warm the milk, put it in a container of warm water or use a bottle warmer. Never use the microwave because milk hotspots can burn your baby's mouth. When you are preparing to feed, swirl the milk in the bottle to blend in the "cream," which will rise to the surface.

If your baby doesn't finish a bottle, you can store the leftovers in the refrigerator for 1 to 2 hours. After that, you will need to discard it because bacteria from your baby's mouth can get into the milk. The live immune cells in your milk keep the bacteria in check in breastmilk from an earlier feed, so it's safe within that 1- to 2-hour window. For more on milk storage, go to KellyMom's excellent summary with all the information you need (Bonyata, 2012).

HOW MUCH MILK DOES MY BABY NEED?

From ages 1 to 6 months, your baby needs approximately 25 ounces per day (Bonyata, 2018a). During growth spurts, that amount may increase a bit, but those times tend to be brief. Unless you are exclusively pumping, you don't need to provide all 25 ounces in pumped milk if your baby is still feeding at the breast. Estimate that your baby needs about 3 ounces per feeding and calculate how many feedings your baby will need when you are apart, with perhaps a bit extra in case you are delayed picking them up.

> *Example:* If baby usually nurses around eight times per day, you can guess that baby might need around 3 ounces per feeding when mom is away (25/8 = 3.1).

This amount is less than what a formula-feed baby needs because a higher percentage of your milk is bioavailable for your baby, so they need less volume to get the same nutrition. When your baby starts solids, your milk is still the primary source of nutrition, but they will consume less breastmilk (14–19 ounces per day).

If your baby is consuming more than this, it could be because the bottle has a fast flow, and their drinking may outpace the cues that say they are full. You might try a nipple with a slower flow. Your baby could also need to suck for comfort (e.g., if they are cutting a tooth). The caregiver may interpret that as hunger. Once the baby has had enough to eat, the caregiver might try a pacifier or teether rather than a bottle to comfort them. Or it could be that your caregiver is thawing too much milk per feed and may be wasting some. Work with your caregiver to ensure that your baby has enough to eat and no milk is wasted. You might also think about freezing some 1-ounce top-up bags so that if you are delayed, your baby can have a snack, but it won't be so much that they don't want to nurse (Needels, 2019). If your baby is taking less milk than expected, it could be because they are reverse cycling and tanking up once you are together again.

REVERSE-CYCLE FEEDING

Some mothers who are separated from their babies during the day find that nighttime parenting becomes super important. It's a time to reconnect with their babies and spend time together. Also, there are some babies who are reluctant to take a bottle even after several months. They tend to take only as much as they minimally need and wait until they are reunited with their mothers to feed, so they do most of their feedings in the middle of the night. When babies get more experienced, they can feed without even waking their mothers. Mothers and babies get lots of contact, and the babies get in many of their daily feeds. Although this method isn't for everyone, some mothers like it (Bonyata, 2018b).

FINDING A BREASTFEEDING-FRIENDLY CHILD CARE PROVIDER

Ideally, your child care provider is breastfeeding friendly. Some are quite willing to learn. The Carolina Global Breastfeeding Institute (n.d.) has free handouts you can download for your child care provider. As you search for a provider, consider a few important things.

- *Do they understand how breastfeeding works?* Do they understand that a breastfed child does not need the same amount of food that a formula-feeding child does?
- *Do they have a place to store your milk, and are they comfortable handling it?* Will they use smaller amounts rather than filling an entire bottle? Breast milk is not a biohazard (as some fear), but it needs to be transferred to a bottle (if it's not already in one) and not contaminated.
- *Are they close enough to your workplace to allow you to drop in and nurse?* This type of arrangement is not always possible, but it can work well (especially if the child care is onsite).

Following are some general considerations you should have when selecting a place for your baby.

- *What is the staff-to-child ratio?* It should not be higher than one staff member for every three babies, with eight infants being the maximum allowed (U.S. Office of Personnel Management, n.d.).

(One mother told me that she made a surprise visit to her child care center only to find her baby screaming in a walker, and she was freezing. She left that day. There was clearly not enough staff, or they didn't care that this baby was cold and upset. Neither explanation is good.) Obviously, the more one-on-one time the staff has with your baby, the better. But beyond staffing, what is their general attitude toward children? That will tell you a lot about how they will act when you are not there.

- *Is there a lot of turnover at the day care center?* This is important to know from an attachment perspective. You want your baby to feel comfortable in your absence, and familiar people will help with that. However, if the center is a revolving door, that can be stressful for your baby.

Full-time day care can be expensive, and some mothers find that alternative work arrangements make more financial sense.

ALTERNATIVE WORK ARRANGEMENTS

A lesson from COVID-19 is that business can be conducted in many creative ways. For many types of jobs, you do not need to be in a traditional office from 8 to 5. For example, could you work at home a couple of days a week? You will still need some child care, but you would be available to nurse and need to pump less often. It's also helpful for maintaining your milk supply. The U.S. Office of Women's Health (2018) also suggests possibly taking Wednesdays off so you can be with your baby and rebuild your supply.

People are asking to reduce work hours for lots of reasons. Caring for aging parents or a child who is having difficulties. Working from home, flexible schedules, and compressed workweeks lead to less traffic in congested areas and are generally better for the environment. These options may seem impossible, but I'd urge you to consider them before ruling them out. If you'd like to do things differently, plan to change things gradually to move to this type of work. It may take weeks or even months, but if you are determined, you can make it happen more often than you might expect.

Flextime and Compressed Work Weeks

"Flextime" refers to starting and finishing work at nonstandard times. It might mean starting early and leaving early or starting late and working later. Compressed workweek is when a full workweek is compressed into four 10-hour days or three 12-hour days. This allows for more full days at home but with full-time benefits.

Part Time

The number of part-time hours can vary tremendously, from a few hours a week to almost full-time. Sometimes employees share their jobs with another person or function as independent contractors who are employed hourly or on a contract basis. Part-time work generally has no benefits, so it's not for everyone, but it may have a higher hourly wage.

Telecommuting

This can be full- or part-time and involves working at home while communicating with your employer via Zoom or similar platforms, telephone, and email. You can telecommute for all or part of your workweek.

Sequencing

Sequencing takes that long view of your life and says you can have it all, but not all at the same time. The idea is that you have a time when you concentrate on your career, then you step out of the work-force for a few years to raise your children.

When your children are in school or are a little more indepen-dent, you return to the workforce. Keep up professional licenses, stay involved in professional organizations, and stay up on your field. While you have young children at home, you might want to limit your workweek to 10 to 15 hours and not take assignments with tight deadlines. That way, you still have the flexibility you need to respond to your children's needs.

Home Full-Time

You may have been employed all your life and now have decided to stay home and focus on the needs of your family. This isn't an option for everyone, but it is something that some women are choosing, even being willing to lower their standard to living to make it happen. In the novel *I Don't Know How She Does It*, Kate Reddy, a career woman with a highly demanding job and two small children, finally decides that she has had enough and has decided to stay home for a while (Pearson, 2002). Kate made a list of her reasons to give up work, which has resonated with many employed mothers:

1. Because I have got two lives and I don't have time to enjoy either of them.
2. Because twenty-four hours are not enough.
3. Because my children will be young for only a short time.
4. Because becoming a man is the waste of a woman.
5. Because I am too tired to think of another reason. (Pearson, 2002, p. 325)

Going from the world of work to home full-time can be a huge culture shock. While at first the change might be a relief, eventually you may long for parts of your old life. Social isolation, the competi-tion among mothers, and the perceived decrease in social standing can all be hard to cope with if you are not prepared for them. Most of these challenges can be overcome, but forewarned is forearmed. Here are some suggestions to help you cope.

First, I recommend that you give yourself at least 6 months until you decide about whether it is working for you. The first 2 to 3 months can be the hardest, but if you hang in there, it usually gets better. Second, get support! Find a group of mothers you enjoy and don't feel like you are in competition with. Women you become friends with during this phase often become lifelong friends. Take the opportunity to do things that renew you but never had the bandwidth for in the past. This can be a great time in your life. Try to make the most of it.

MAKING WORK WORK FOR YOU

You may decide that you still need or want to continue working, but you don't like your present job. The early days of blending your work self with your mother self can be challenging. Before changing jobs, consider what it is that you don't like in your current situation. There may be a way that you can make a change in the job you have. Or you may need something different, with more flexibility. You need to advocate for yourself and your baby to get the accommodations that you need. Work is changing. We learned a lot during the lockdown. Employers learned that not everyone needs to be in the office to do their work. Employees learned the same thing. This is a great time to ask for what you want. As you're considering your options, think about what you would love to have in a job. Don't cut off possibilities quite yet. You can be realistic later.

Imagine Your Ideal Job

Families have made many creative choices about work, including different shifts, fathers or nongestational mothers home full-time, and both partners working part time. Take a moment and think about what your ideal life would look like. In your ideal life, what type of work and how much of it would you do? How would you get to and from work? What type of child care arrangements would you make (including staying home yourself)? It's hard to make changes if you don't know what your ultimate goal is.

Realistically Assess How Much You Are Netting Now

How much are you netting in your current job? When you calculate all of the hidden expenses, you might find that it's actually costing you to work. You might net the same, or even more, with a part-time job. You do have to also consider the cost of losing your benefits and retirement. Those are not insignificant. After you've calculated everything, remember, it's not how much you make; it's how much you get to keep. Also, consider whether you can live on less. One of my favorite books on this is *The Complete Tightwad Gazette: Promoting Thrift as a Viable Alternative Lifestyle* (Dacyzyn, 1998). Cutting expenses expands your options. And if you want to have a greener lifestyle, cutting expenses, especially in the way *Tightwad Gazette* recommends, will allow you to do that too.

Develop a Plan

If you want a livable working arrangement, you will have to take the initiative. Thinking back to what you want for an ideal job, research your options and present a plan. Try to anticipate your employer's concerns and tell them how you will address them. Realistically, you may need to change employers to get what you want, but don't jump to that option without thinking everything through.

Don't Rush Into Change

Your plan is more likely to succeed if it's not made on impulse. Cautionary tales abound of men and women leaving their high-powered jobs to open a little store or country inn—only to be miserable in their new lives. You'll be happier with your new arrangement if you've had some time to think it through and weigh your many possible options.

Be Confident

You may feel a bit out of sorts because your life has changed so much. But you haven't lost any of your abilities. In fact, you've expanded them. Be confident that you have unique skills to offer and honest about your needs and limitations. Realize too that not everyone will be willing to make these types of accommodations. If they don't, talk to someone else. Remember, breastfeeding accommodations are a right, not a favor. And work accommodations are something that an increasing number of families want. More and more families want work–life balance. There's never been a better time to think about how you could work differently.

CONCLUSION

Combining breastfeeding with employment can take some trial and error before you have the right balance. Many mothers have walked this path before you. Recognize what you need, be confident in asking for it, and plan as much as you can. This phase of life may seem particularly intense, but every bit of breastfeeding you do is good for you and your baby. I wish you success in working through your unique arrangements.

CHAPTER 18

WHEN FEEDING AT THE BREAST ISN'T AN OPTION

It is a sad thing when a mother decides she has to close the door to her nursing experience or desire for a breastfeeding experience. I've seen enough moms come to peace with their decisions that I can counsel other moms that surely, they too will get through the loss. It may be the only option left. It may be the right decision.... But—and I think it's a big but—don't avoid acknowledging the loss and disappointment. She may not understand why this outcome was part of her journey in life.... But we know that the way she honors her heart is naming the loss.

—Chris Auer (2021, p. 59)

Social media campaigns often argue that mothers are pressured to breastfeed, which can be a disaster for them when it doesn't work. Is breastfeeding promotion the problem or is it the lack of support for mothers? Even on my brief breastfeeding survey, I had comments like this one: "I am a three-time failed breastfeeder." Comments like that make me want to rail against our current system. What happens when mothers want to breastfeed and can't? A study from the United Kingdom found that mothers who intended to breastfeed and did not had higher rates of depression than mothers who intended to breastfeed and were able to (Borra et al., 2015). They used data from the Avon Longitudinal Study of Parents and Children, which included 14,541 pregnancies in Avon, England.

A study from the U.S. Centers for Disease Control and Prevention had similar findings. They found that women who breastfed for more than 8 weeks had the lowest rate of postpartum depression (11.8%). In contrast, women who breastfed for less than 8 weeks had the highest rate (15.6%). Women who never breastfed were in the middle (14%; Bauman et al., 2020). These findings were based on data from 31 sites and included 32,659 women. They show the protective effect of breastfeeding when it's going well, and also what happens when it isn't.

WHY MOTHERS STOP

Mothers stop breastfeeding before they want to for many reasons. This often happens in the first few weeks. Here are some of the most common reasons.

Pain

Pain with no help is a common reason for stopping. Being in toe-curling pain for days and weeks will wreak havoc on mental health. Unfortunately, in the absence of help, stopping is the logical choice. We are not serving mothers well here.

Recurring Infections

Sometimes mothers stop because they have recurring infections such as mastitis or thrush. Infections can be painful, and their recurrence disheartening. Some mothers have even gotten abscesses, which had to be surgically drained. Although you can continue breastfeeding through that, many mothers feel traumatized by the experience and don't want to continue.

Low Milk Supply

Some mothers stop because of low milk supply. It could be that there was an injury to the breast or insufficient glandular tissue (IGT), which made it impossible to bring in a full supply, or it could be that breast-feeding was not managed well in the first few weeks when mothers were setting their milk production. Some mothers can bring in a full supply even after getting off to a dismal start, but it is exceptionally difficult to do that. A mother in our survey described how IGT, tongue-tie, and lack of help made breastfeeding impossible.

> My birth was relatively fast . . . and straightforward, but I was given Pitocin right after delivering my placenta as the doctor was not comfortable with the blood loss he was witnessing. My baby was with me for an hour or so, then taken away. It was not possible to room in, so I was called into the nursery whenever she woke up hungry, but I was given no assistance whatsoever. I was discharged 2 days later and by day 5 baby was severely jaundiced and dehydrated. I later discovered she had a posterior tongue tie, a lip tie, and I have IGT. I was never able to breastfeed exclusively, but I managed to provide about 75% of her needs through pumping, herbs, and using a LactAid.

Mothers may also believe that they have a low supply and start supplementing. Industry preys on their fears. Although formula companies make a useful product, they are no friend to breastfeeding. They make money when breastfeeding fails and will send you home with a coupon for their product "just in case." More supplementation means fewer breast emptyings, which leads to low milk supply.

Difficult Birth

The type of birth you had, along with medications, epidurals, and prolonged separation, can all make early breastfeeding difficult. Traumatic births can also delay lactogenesis II, which can lead to jaundice and dehydration, as this mother described:

> In the end I was unable to breastfeed traditionally and had to instead exclusively pump which was VERY difficult. This was

293

due to a combination of factors including a traumatic birth (for mom and baby), inverted nipples, my being drugged afterwards due to c-section, not being prepared (despite thinking I was), and not receiving the guidance I believe that I should have in the hospital. I am 12 months postpartum and still cry every time I think about my failure to breastfeed my child traditionally. I know that [breastfed] is best and I am proud to have supplied him with breastmilk for 7 months but it still makes me incredibly sad.

Prolonged Separation of Mother and Baby

If your baby was premature, ill, or hospitalized, prolonged separations may have affected your milk production during a crucial phase. If you delivered in a hospital that supports breastfeeding, you might have been told to pump to protect your supply. However, some hospitals do not support breastfeeding. One of our local hospitals inexplicably does not allow parents to even hold their babies in the neonatal intensive care unit, making breastfeeding close to impossible.

Early Return to Work and Lack of Workplace Support

Breastfeeding can also be compromised when mothers return to work right away. This happens more often in the United States, where 25% of new mothers are back at work by 2 weeks postpartum (Lukas, 2019). Lack of workplace support also makes it difficult to sustain breastfeeding, as this mother from our survey described. Even with all the obstacles, she still breastfed for 4 months, which is amazing.

I was 20 and healthy; I wasn't even in the hospital for a full 24 hours from check-in to discharge and my family doctor was the one who caught my baby. She made me feel empowered during my birth, which helped with my confidence. I received WIC support and had a First Steps nurse come to our house. . . . I was poor and states away from home and family. I went back to working full time when my daughter was 2 weeks old. Where I worked was a secure building and the only room that was private was the rest rooms, so I would use a manual pump while sitting on the toilet; it was hard. I only breastfed for about 4 months and I feel like with more support/knowledge I would have done it for much longer. I remember one of the only times I fed her in public was while standing in line at a food bank, the process of standing in line had taken much longer than I had anticipated or planned for. Overall, I feel sad that I didn't "stick with it" but I am happy that I did my best with what resources and tools I had at the time.

BREASTFEEDING GRIEF

All lactation consultants hear stories of sadness and sorrow around breastfeeding. U.K. psychologist Dr. Amy Brown has conducted the most research on this topic, and she summarized it in her book, *Why Breastfeeding Grief and Trauma Matter* (Brown, 2019). She noted that women who started breastfeeding and stopped before they were ready experienced a whole range of emotions: grief, anger, guilt, shame, and frustration. One mother in her book described her experience of not being able to nurse her third child. Although she was able to pump and provide her milk, she missed the physical contact and the relationship part of it. Even after nursing her first two babies and helping other mothers to breastfeed, she noted:

> I felt like I never wanted to hear the word again, much less have anything to do with anyone who still inhabited that world. I didn't want the reminder that, this time, the oh-so-natural process just wasn't working, that my dear little baby was being so thoroughly failed by his mother. Feeding had become a simple transaction: empty baby plus full bottle equals full baby. And it wasn't a transaction that I wanted; it was a relationship. Because for me, breastfeeding wasn't just about getting milk

into my baby. It was so much more than that; it was the quiet moments holding my baby in my arms at the end of the day, the cheeky trying to talk with their mouth full, mischief eyes looking up at me, the patting to say which side they wanted first, sitting up post-feed and saying, "Yum!" and all the other skin-to-skin moments that were so important to bonding. (Brown, 2019, pp. 14–15)

Brown (2019) noted that mothers feel that they've missed out on breastfeeding as a mothering tool, and not being able to do it can cause them to question their own identities as mothers. Breastfeeding can also be a source of healing when there has been a difficult birth, or the baby is sick or premature. Mothers' feelings about breastfeeding and not being able to do it are complex and tied up in identity and culture—for example, Cammie Goldhammer described the impact of breastfeeding in Native communities in the United States:

When indigenous people breastfeed their babies, they are reclaiming their traditional practices, which not only has the power to change the life course of future generations but heal those that came before us. (Cited in Brown, 2019, p. 24)

Similarly, Kimberly Seals Allers described the importance of breastfeeding in American Black communities:

Black breastfeeding is a revolutionary act, an act of resistance in and of itself. When Black women breastfeed, they are reversing narratives, reclaiming traditions that were taken from them, countering stereotypes, and reestablishing the infant-feeding norm in our communities. (Cited in Brown, 2019, pp. 24–25)

Dr. Brown concluded her discussion about the meaning that women ascribe to breastfeeding with the following observation. I think it gets at the heart of why women grieve when they cannot breastfeed; telling them to "just give a bottle" doesn't help.

Yes, despite all this depth and complexity of belief and feeling, women are increasingly told that formula milk is a comparable substitute for breastfeeding. And to argue otherwise judges them or is anti-feminist. While formula may feed the baby, women's desire to have their bodies work does not go away because they can formula-feed. Women's feeling that their body has let them down does not go away because they can formula-feed. Women's desire to mother in the way they want does not go away because they can formula-feed. (Brown, 2019, pp. 32–33)

Brown (2019) found that the length of breastfeeding did not increase the risk of depression, but whether a mother was ready to stop did. Mothers who stopped breastfeeding because of pain, physical difficulty, or lack of support were more likely to be depressed. If they wanted to stop because they were ready, their risk of depression was substantially less.

If breastfeeding mothers are depressed, practitioners and family members alike often tell them to stop to make it all better. Mothers often see this quite differently and have told me that "breastfeeding is the only thing that is going well for me," as this mother in Brown's study described:

I hated my life and I hated myself. I thought I was a terrible, useless mother apart from breastfeeding, that was the one thing that I was getting right. Why did everyone want to take that away from me? (Brown, 2019, p. 54)

TAKING CARE OF YOURSELF IF YOU CAN'T BREASTFEED

As Amy Brown's research shows, many women grieve the loss of breastfeeding when they cannot do it or cannot do it for as long as they want. If this has happened to you, it's important that you acknowledge that grief and work through it. In some cases, you may want to talk with a counselor or someone who can help process your feelings of grief and loss. Your feelings matter, and others shouldn't minimize them. Yes, you can feed your baby another way, but you have lost something as well.

If you were given bad advice that caused breastfeeding to fail, you may have difficulty letting go of your sadness because it was *preventable*. I'd encourage you to join a support group or talk to a counselor who can help you process your feelings or write about them, as writing can help you resolve traumatic feelings. I'd also encourage you to let yourself off the hook. You did the best you could with the information you had.

Your anger may be tougher to resolve because your breastfeeding problems and the suffering they caused didn't have to happen. I completely understand why you are mad, but I am urging you not to stay there. Anger will eventually eat at you and keep you from moving forward. Processing your anger by writing about it or talking to a counselor, can help you let it go. You can also channel it in a positive direction. I've known many breastfeeding peer supporters, lactation consultants, and doulas who have turned their own bad experiences into a catalyst for change for other women. But your own mental health will be better if you can let this go before you launch into a new area of work.

During this time of grief, you might want to avoid breastfeeding social media and even limit your exposure to nursing mothers until you feel less vulnerable. It's okay to do what you need to protect yourself. At some point, you may be comfortable being around nursing mothers, but if being around them makes you feel bad, it's okay to step back. Breastfeeding is only one part of being a mother. You have not lost your relationship with your baby, and you have not lost your ability to form a secure attachment—the most important thing.

THE IMPORTANCE OF ATTACHMENT

When you are in the midst of the crisis, or even years after the fact, you might feel that all is lost, that the loss of breastfeeding has tainted your whole parenting experience with sorrow. Against this backdrop, I want to bring you some hope. As I said in Chapter 1, *attachment supersedes breastfeeding as a parenting goal.* If there is one variable that predicts later success in life, it's a secure attachment. It predicts achievement in school and positive relationships. It builds resilience in children to weather the storms of life, which is significantly related to their long-term health (Puig et al., 2013; Schore, 2001).

Your baby can have a secure attachment to you even if you are not breastfeeding. In fact, much of the early research on attachment was done when the majority of families were formula-feeding. **Attachment is not the consolation prize; it's *the* prize.** Breastfeeding facilitates secure attachment, but it is not the only way to get there.

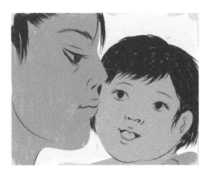

The most important thing is having a positive relationship with your baby. You can have that even if you are not breastfeeding.

To facilitate a secure attachment, Drs. Mary Ainsworth and John Bowlby (1991) identified two important things in the last article they wrote together. John Bowlby was the British psychiatrist whose name is synonymous with attachment research. Mary Ainsworth was his American counterpart who developed the measure of attachment. This is what they identified as critical to developing a secure attachment: maternal/caregiver proximity and responsive care. You're near your baby, and you respond to them when they cry. Note that they did not mention breastfeeding as a prerequisite for attachment. Here are some examples of how you can facilitate that.

Using a Supplementer

If mothers do not have a full supply, or even if they have no supply at all, many choose to feed their babies at the breast using a supplementer.

You can buy a special device, such as the supplemental nursing system, or you can make your own with 5-gauge tubing and a bottle. (Use "5-gauge silicone medical tubing" in your search, or you'll get a lot of plumbing supplies.)

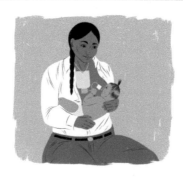

With a supplemental nursing system, your baby receives supplemental nutrition while at your breast.

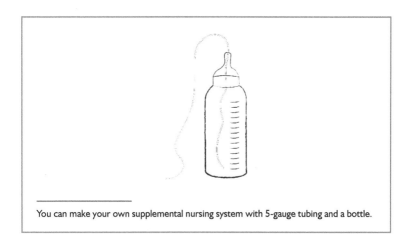

You can make your own supplemental nursing system with 5-gauge tubing and a bottle.

The principle is that while your baby is suckling at your breast, they are also being fed with a small tube that delivers formula or expressed breastmilk to them. These devices can be used to help mothers increase their supply by having their babies at the breast; the breast is stimulated, and babies are receiving supplementary nutrition. It can also be used by mothers who want to feed their baby at the breast, even when there is no milk. This technique can also be used by adoptive or nongestational mothers. (For advice on how to do this, I'd recommend Alyssa Schnell's, 2013, *Breastfeeding Without Birthing*.) This can be a permanent way to feed or a stepping stone to bringing in a full supply (Ruddle, 2021).

This supplement system works well for many mothers, but others have a love–hate relationship with their supplementer. They find the process cumbersome, and they feel that they can't do this when they are out and about. Other mothers may wonder why you don't "just use a bottle."

Mothers who use a supplementer enjoy the physical contact with their babies, with the baby gazing up into their eyes while feeding at the breast. This technique is also useful when babies are too small

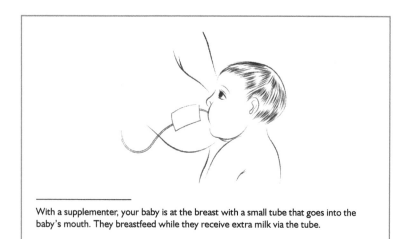

With a supplementer, your baby is at the breast with a small tube that goes into the baby's mouth. They breastfeed while they receive extra milk via the tube.

to have a full feeding at the breast and need the help of a supplement to make sure that they are getting enough to eat before they tire out. You can use your own pumped milk, donor milk (discussed next), or formula.

Donor Milk

Sometimes mothers (and some dads) opt to use donor milk to feed their babies instead of using formula. If your baby is term, you usually cannot get milk from milk banks as their supply is for preterm and hospitalized babies. Some mothers use networks of informal milk sharing. This is where breastfeeding mothers pump and offer their milk to a mother (or dad) who wants to feed their baby human milk.

Informal milk sharing is controversial among practitioners in the breastfeeding world. Medical practitioners, in particular, discourage this practice. Other practitioners know that this happens but turn the other way or even actively encourage it. The practitioners who discourage it worry about possible contamination, infectious diseases, or mothers adding things to their milk to stretch it out (Sriraman et al., 2018). (The temptation to add things seems to be more of a problem when mothers pay for the milk rather than when it is donated.) The concerns about contamination or possible infection are legitimate, so if you decide to go this route, I'd encourage due diligence. Get a health history from the mother who is donating. Some mothers get milk from someone they know. Do not ever pay for milk because that is when you are more likely to run into problems. I'd recommend that you go to EatsonFeets (https://www.eatsonfeets.org/), a site that facilitates milk sharing and has been around since 2010.

Paced Bottle-Feeding

Paced bottle-feeding is a way to "feed with love and respect" (Nicholson & Parker, 2019). Who controls how much the baby eats is one key difference between breast and bottle-feeding. With breastfeeding, babies control how much they eat. With bottle-feeding, the adult does. It is easy for babies to eat too much with a bottle. Bottle-fed babies constantly have their satiety cues (the cues that tell them they are full) overridden by their caretakers, which has consequences. In one study, when older babies were given a bottle or cup and allowed to feed themselves, exclusively bottle-fed babies were more likely to finish the full amount rather than stopping when they are full (Li et al., 2010). It's one theory why bottle-feeding may increase the risk of obesity in childhood.

To counter that, you can pace bottle-feeding. Sit your baby more upright than they would be while breastfeeding; they can still be close to your body. If they are upright, gravity does not keep pouring milk into their mouths. They need to be able to stop and start.

Be sure to feed your baby on both sides of your body because gazing up at you helps with their eye development. Be sure to spend time cuddling and looking into their eyes. This is when you can

303

connect with your baby; you can even have your baby skin-to-skin while bottle-feeding them. When your baby is full, stop—even if you still have milk left in the bottle. If you are feeding with formula and are worried about wasting it, try mixing up smaller amounts. You can always make more. That way, your baby still gets enough to eat, but you don't feel like you are throwing away tons of formula.

Babywearing

Babywearing is another way that you can connect with your baby. There are dozens of great carriers on the market. For young infants, I prefer a baby sling that goes diagonally across your body. These types of carriers are easier on your back and shoulders, and you can keep your baby close to you. You will still need one hand on your baby in the carrier, but these allow you to be up and about while still keeping your baby calm.

Baby carriers also help with attachment. One of the most elegant studies I've seen on this was published way back in 1990 (Anisfeld et al., 1990). The authors randomly assigned mothers who were at high risk for child abuse to have either a soft carrier or a car-seat carrier for their babies. None of these mothers were breastfeeding. They found that mothers who had soft carriers were more responsive to their babies at 3 months. By 12 to 18 months, when attachment is measured, these babies were more likely to have a secure attachment compared with babies who were in car-seat-type carriers.

Infant Massage

Massaging your baby is good for both of you and releases oxytocin because of the oxytocin receptors in the palm of the hand (Uvnäs Moberg, 2013). Many studies with preterm infants have shown that massage turns off their stress system and allows them to grow. Use

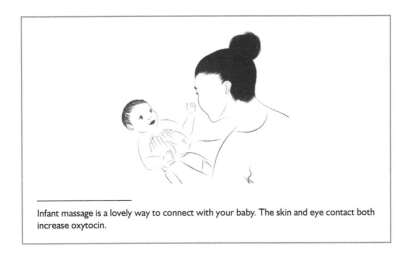

Infant massage is a lovely way to connect with your baby. The skin and eye contact both increase oxytocin.

lotion or corn starch so that your hands glide over your baby's skin. Use broad strokes toward your baby's core while looking into their eyes. It's a great way to connect and can help you overcome the stresses of the early weeks.

CONCLUSION

If you've lost breastfeeding, you may feel anger, sorrow, deep grief, and even symptoms of trauma. These feelings are real, but breastfeeding is only one part of the amazing journey of motherhood. Acknowledge that you feel bad about what happened, but recognize that you still have many other ways to connect with your baby. The real goal is to form a secure attachment to your baby. A secure attachment gets your baby through life and allows them to be the person they are meant to be (Nicholson & Parker, 2019; Owenz, 2021; Schore, 2001). If you and your baby form a secure attachment, mothering will be more enjoyable for you both because it's a relationship—you and your baby will be set for life.

REFERENCES

Abramowitz, J. S., Schwartz, S. A., Moore, K. M., & Luenzmann, K. R. (2003). Obsessive-compulsive symptoms in pregnancy and the puerperium: A review of the literature. *Journal of Anxiety Disorders, 17*(4), 461–478. https://doi.org/10.1016/s0887-6185(02)00206-2

Adedinsewo, D. A., Fleming, A. S., Steiner, M., Meaney, M. J., Girard, A. W., & the MAVAN team. (2014). Maternal anxiety and breastfeeding: Findings from the MAVAN (Maternal Adversity, Vulnerability and Neurodevelopment) Study. *Journal of Human Lactation, 30*(1), 102–109. https://doi.org/10.1177/0890334413504244

Ainsworth, M. D. S., & Bowlby, J. (1991). An ethological approach to personality development. *American Psychologist, 46*(4), 333–341. https://doi.org/10.1037/0003-066X.46.4.333

Alcorn, K. L., O'Donovan, A., Patrick, J. C., Creedy, D., & Devilly, G. J. (2010). A prospective longitudinal study of the prevalence of post-traumatic stress disorder resulting from childbirth events. *Psychological Medicine, 40*(11), 1849–1859. https://doi.org/10.1017/S0033291709992224

American Academy of Pediatrics. (2016). SIDS and other sleep-related infant deaths: Updated 2016 recommendations for a safe infant sleeping environment. *Pediatrics, 138*(5), 320162938. https://doi.org/10.1542/peds.2016-2938

American Academy of Pediatrics Task Force on Sudden Infant Death Syndrome. (2005). The changing concept of sudden infant death syndrome: Diagnostic coding shifts, controversies regarding the sleeping environment, and new variables to consider in reducing risk. *Pediatrics, 116*(5), 1245–1255. https://doi.org/10.1542/peds.2005-1499

American Academy of Pediatrics Task Force on Sudden Infant Death Syndrome. (2011a). Policy Statement: SIDS and other sleep-related infant deaths: Expansion of recommendations for a safe infant sleeping environment. *Pediatrics*, *128*(5), 1030–1039. https://doi.org/10.1542/peds.2011-2284

American Academy of Pediatrics Task Force on Sudden Infant Death Syndrome. (2011b). Technical Report: SIDS and other sleep-related infant deaths: Expansion of recommendations for a safe infant sleeping environment. *Pediatrics*, *128*(5), e1341–e1367. https://doi.org/10.1542/peds.2011-2285

American Psychiatric Association. (2013). *Diagnostic and statistical manual of mental disorders* (5th ed.).

Anghelescu, I. G., Kohnen, R., Szegedi, A., Klement, S., & Kieser, M. (2006). Comparison of Hypericum extract WS 5570 and paroxetine in ongoing treatment after recovery from an episode of moderate to severe depression: Results from a randomized multicenter study. *Pharmacopsychiatry*, *39*(6), 213–219. https://doi.org/10.1055/s-2006-951388

Anisfeld, E., Casper, V., Nozyce, M., & Cunningham, N. (1990). Does infant carrying promote attachment? An experimental study of the effects of increased physical contact on the development of attachment. *Child Development*, *61*(5), 1617–1627. https://doi.org/10.2307/1130769

Ansara, D., Cohen, M. M., Gallop, R., Kung, R., & Schei, B. (2005). Predictors of women's physical health problems after childbirth. *Journal of Psychosomatic Obstetrics and Gynaecology*, *26*(2), 115–125. https://doi.org/10.1080/01443610400023064

Audelo, L. (2013). *The virtual breastfeeding culture: Seeking mother-to-mother support in the digital age*. Praeclarus Press.

Auer, C. (2021). *A lullaby: Reflections for caregivers of breastfeeding families*. Praeclarus Press.

Babyak, M., Blumenthal, J. A., Herman, S., Khatri, P., Doraiswamy, M., Moore, K., Craighead, W. E., Baldewicz, T. T., & Krishnan, K. R. (2000). Exercise treatment for major depression: Maintenance of therapeutic benefit at 10 months. *Psychosomatic Medicine*, *62*(5), 633–638. https://doi.org/10.1097/00006842-200009000-00006

Ball, H. (2006). Parent–infant bed-sharing behavior: Effects of feeding type and presence of father. *Human Nature*, *17*(3), 301–318. https://doi.org/10.1007/s12110-006-1011-1

Ball, H. L. (2007). Bed-sharing practices of initially breastfed infants in the first 6 months of life. *Infant and Child Development, 16*(4), 387–401. https://doi.org/10.1002/icd.519

Bascom, E. M., & Napolitano, M. A. (2016). Breastfeeding duration and primary reasons for breastfeeding cessation among women with post-partum depressive symptoms. *Journal of Human Lactation, 32*(2), 282–291. https://doi.org/10.1177/0890334415619908

Bauman, B. L., Ko, J. Y., Cox, S., D'Angelo Mph, D. V., Warner, L., Folger, S., Tevendale, H. D., Coy, K. C., Harrison, L., & Barfield, W. D. (2020). Postpartum depressive symptoms and provider discussions about peri-natal depression: United States 2018. *Morbidity & Mortality Weekly Report, 69*(19), 575–581. https://doi.org/10.15585/mmwr.mm6919a2

Beck, C. T. (2004). Birth trauma: In the eye of the beholder. *Nursing Research, 53*(1), 28–35. https://doi.org/10.1097/00006199-200401000-00005

Beck, C. T. (2011). A metaethnography of traumatic childbirth and its after-math: Amplifying causal looping. *Qualitative Health Research, 21*(3), 301–311. https://doi.org/10.1177/1049732310390698

Beck, C. T., Gable, R. K., Sakala, C., & Declercq, E. R. (2011). Post-traumatic stress disorder in new mothers: Results from a two-stage U.S. national survey. *Birth, 38*(3), 216–227. https://doi.org/10.1111/j.1523-536X.2011.00475.x

Beck, C. T., & Watson, S. (2008). Impact of birth trauma on breast-feeding: A tale of two pathways. *Nursing Research, 57*(4), 228–236. https://doi.org/10.1097/01.NNR.0000313494.87282.90

Benedict, M. I., Paine, L., & Paine, L. (1994). *Long-term effects of child sexual abuse on functioning in pregnancy and pregnancy outcomes (final report).* National Center of Child Abuse & Neglect.

Berg-Drazin, P. (2019). IBCLCs and craniosacral therapists: Strange bed-fellows or perfect match. In K. A. Kendall-Tackett (Ed.), *Breast and nipple pain II* (pp. 37–59). Praeclarus Press.

Bergink, V., Gibney, S. M., & Drexhage, H. A. (2014). Autoimmunity, inflam-mation, and psychosis: A search for peripheral markers. *Biological Psychiatry, 75*(4), 324–331. https://doi.org/10.1016/j.biopsych.2013.09.037

Blair, P. S., & Ball, H. L. (2004). The prevalence and characteristics asso-ciated with parent-infant bed-sharing in England. *Archives of Disease in Childhood, 89*(12), 1106–1110. https://doi.org/10.1136/adc.2003.038067

Blair, P. S., Ball, H. L., McKenna, J. J., Feldman-Winter, L., Marinelli, K. A., Bartick, M. C., Young, M., Noble, L., Calhoun, S., Elliott-Rudder, M., Kair, L. R., Lappin, S., Larson, I., Lawrence, R. A., Lefort, Y., Marshall, N., Mitchell, K., Murak, C., Myers, E., Reece-Stretman, S., Rosen-Carole, C., Rotehnberg, S., Schmidt, T., Seo, T., Sriraman, N., Stehel, E. K., Wight, N., Wonodi, A., & the Academy of Breastfeeding Medicine. (2020). Bedsharing and breastfeeding: The Academy of Breastfeeding Medicine Protocol #6, Revision 2019. *Breastfeeding Medicine*, *15*(1), 5–16. https://doi.org/10.1089/bfm.2019.29144.psb

Blair, P. S., Heron, J., & Fleming, P. J. (2010). Relationship between bed sharing and breastfeeding: Longitudinal, population-based analysis. *Pediatrics*, *126*(5), e1119–e1126. https://doi.org/10.1542/peds.2010-1277

Blair, P. S., Sidebotham, P., Berry, P. J., Evans, M., & Fleming, P. J. (2006). Major epidemiological changes in sudden infant death syndrome: A 20-year population-based study in the UK. *The Lancet*, *367*(9507), 314–319. https://doi.org/10.1016/S0140-6736(06)67968-3

Blumenthal, J. A., Babyak, M. A., Doraiswamy, P. M., Watkins, L., Hoffman, B. M., Barbour, K. A., Herman, S., Craighead, W. E., Brosse, A. L., Waugh, R., Hinderliter, A., & Sherwood, A. (2007). Exercise and pharmacotherapy in the treatment of major depressive disorder. *Psychosomatic Medicine*, *69*(7), 587–596. https://doi.org/10.1097/PSY.0b013e318148c19a

Bonyata, K. (2012). *Human milk storage.* https://kellymom.com/store/freehandouts/milkstorage01.pdf

Bonyata, K. (2018a). *How much expressed milk will my baby need?* https://kellymom.com/bf/pumpingmoms/pumping/milkcalc

Bonyata, K. (2018b). *Reverse cycling.* https://kellymom.com/bf/normal/reverse-cycling

Borra, C., Iacovou, M., & Sevilla, A. (2015). New evidence on breastfeeding and postpartum depression: The importance of understanding women's intentions. *Maternal and Child Health Journal*, *19*(4), 897–907. https://doi.org/10.1007/s10995-014-1591-z

Brown, A. E. (2016). *Breastfeeding uncovered: Who really decides how we feed our babies?* Pinter & Martin.

Brown, A. E. (2019). *Why breastfeeding grief and trauma matter.* Pinter & Martin.

Buser, G. L., Mató, S., Zhang, A. Y., Metcalf, B. J., Beall, B., & Thomas, A. R. (2017). Notes from the field: Late-onset infant Group B streptococcus infection associated with maternal consumption of capsules containing dehydrated placenta—Oregon, 2016. *Morbidity & Mortality Weekly Report, 66*(25), 677–678. https://doi.org/10.15585/mmwr.mm6625a4

Buss, C., Davis, E. P., Shahbaba, B., Pruessner, J. C., Head, K., & Sandman, C. A. (2012). Maternal cortisol over the course of pregnancy and subsequent child amygdala and hippocampus volumes and affective problems. *Proceedings of the National Academy of Sciences of the United States of America, 109*(20), E1312–E1319. https://doi.org/10.1073/pnas.1201295109

Buttner, M. M., Brock, R. L., O'Hara, M. W., & Stuart, S. (2015). Efficacy of yoga for depressed postpartum women: A randomized controlled trial. *Complementary Therapies in Clinical Practice, 21*(2), 94–100. https://doi.org/10.1016/j.ctcp.2015.03.003

Bystrova, K., Widström, A. M., Matthiesen, A. S., Ransjö-Arvidson, A.-B., Welles-Nyström, B., Wassberg, C., Vorontsov, I., & Uvnäs-Moberg, K. (2003). Skin-to-skin contact may reduce negative consequences of "the stress of being born": A study on temperature in newborn infants, subjected to different ward routines in St. Petersburg. *Acta Paediatrica, 92*(3), 320–326. https://doi.org/10.1111/j.1651-2227.2003.tb00553.x

California Breastfeeding Coalition. (n.d.). *Workplace lactation accommodation/ Paid family leave.* https://californiabreastfeeding.org/focus-areas/workplaces/

Cappelletti, M., Della Bella, S., Ferrazzi, E., Mavilio, D., & Divanovic, S. (2016). Inflammation and preterm birth. *Journal of Leukocyte Biology, 99*(1), 67–78. https://doi.org/10.1189/jlb.3MR0615-272RR

Carolina Global Breastfeeding Institute. (n.d.). *CGBI: Ten steps to breastfeeding-friendly child care.* https://sph.unc.edu/cgbi/ten-steps-to-breastfeeding-friendly-child-care/

Cassar-Uhl, D. (2014). *Finding sufficiency: Breastfeeding with insufficient glandular tissue.* Praeclarus Press.

Centers for Disease Control and Prevention. (2020a). *Breastfeeding report card.* https://www.cdc.gov/breastfeeding/data/reportcard.htm

Centers for Disease Control and Prevention. (2020b). *Postpartum depression.* https://www.cdc.gov/reproductivehealth/depression/index.htm#Postpartum

Cheyney, M., Henning, M., Horan, H., Bovbjerg, M. L., & Ferguson, M. (2019a). From policy to practice: Women's experiences of breast-feeding-friendly workplaces, Part 1. *Clinical Lactation, 10*(3), 104–112. https://doi.org/10.1891/2158-0782.10.3.104

Cheyney, M., Henning, M., Horan, H., Bovbjerg, M. L., & Ferguson, M. (2019b). From policy to practice: Women's experiences of breast-feeding-friendly worksites, Part 2. *Clinical Lactation, 10*(3), 113–120. https://doi.org/10.1891/2158-0782.10.3.113

Coentro, V. S., Perrella, S. L., Lai, C. T., Rea, A., Dymock, M., & Geddes, D. T. (2021). Nipple shield use does not impact sucking dynamics in breastfeeding infants of mothers with nipple pain. *European Journal of Pediatrics, 180*(5), 1537–1543. https://doi.org/10.1007/s00431-020-03901-3

Cole, M. (2014). Placenta medicine as a galactogogue: Tradition or trend? *Clinical Lactation, 5*(4), 116–122. https://doi.org/10.1891/2158-0782. 5.4.116

Coles, J., Anderson, A., & Loxton, D. (2016). Breastfeeding duration after childhood sexual abuse: An Australian cohort study. *Journal of Human Lactation, 32*(3), NP28–NP35. https://doi.org/10.1177/ 0890334415590782

Colson, S. (2019). *Biological nurturing: Instinctual breastfeeding* (rev. ed.). Praeclarus Press.

Cooney, G. M., Dwan, K., Grieg, C. A., Lawlor, D. A., Rimer, J., Waugh, F. R., McMurdo, M., & Mead, G. E. (2013). Exercise for depression. *Cochrane Database of Systematic Reviews, 12*. https://doi.org/10.1002/14651858. CD004366.pub6

Cotterman, K. J. (2004). Reverse pressure softening: A simple tool to prepare areola for easier latching during engorgement. *Journal of Human Lactation, 20*(2), 227–237. https://doi.org/10.1177/0890334404264224

Cox, S. (2010). A case of dysphoric milk-ejection reflex (D-MER). *Breastfeeding Review, 18*(1), 16–18.

Dacyzyn, A. (1998). *The complete tightwad gazette: Promoting thrift as a viable alternative lifestyle.* Villard.

Danese, A., Moffitt, T. E., Harrington, H., Milne, B. J., Polanczyk, G., Pariante, C. M., Poulton, R., & Caspi, A. (2009). Adverse childhood experiences and adult risk factors for age-related disease: Depression, inflammation, and clustering of metabolic risk markers. *Archives of*

Pediatrics & Adolescent Medicine, 163(12), 1135–1143. https://doi.org/10.1001/archpediatrics.2009.214

Davidson, E. L., & Ollerton, R. L. (2020). Partner behaviours improving breastfeeding outcomes: An integrative review. *Women and Birth: Journal of the Australian College of Midwives, 33*(1), e15–e23. https://doi.org/10.1016/j.wombi.2019.05.010

Deligiannidis, K. M., & Freeman, M. P. (2010). Complementary and alternative medicine for the treatment of depressive disorders in women. *The Psychiatric Clinics of North America, 33*(2), 441–463. https://doi.org/10.1016/j.psc.2010.01.002

Dennis, C.-L., Grigoriadis, S., Zupancic, J., Kiss, A., & Ravitz, P. (2020). Telephone-based nurse-delivered interpersonal psychotherapy for postpartum depression: Nationwide randomised controlled trial. *The British Journal of Psychiatry, 216*(4), 189–196. https://doi.org/10.1192/bjp.2019.275

Dewey, K. G., Nommsen-Rivers, L. A., Heinig, M. J., & Cohen, R. J. (2003). Risk factors for suboptimal infant breastfeeding behavior, delayed onset of lactation, and excess neonatal weight loss. *Pediatrics, 112*(3 Pt. 1), 607–619. https://doi.org/10.1542/peds.112.3.607

Diego, M. A., Field, T., Jones, N. A., & Hernandez-Reif, M. (2006). Withdrawn and intrusive maternal interaction style and infant frontal EEG asymmetry shifts in infants of depressed and non-depressed mothers. *Infant Behavior and Development, 29*(2), 220–229. https://doi.org/10.1016/j.infbeh.2005.12.002

DiTomasso, D., Wambach, K. A., Roberts, M. B., Erickson-Owens, D. A., Quigley, A., & Newbury, J. M. (2022). Maternal worry about infant weight and its influence on artificial milk supplementation and breastfeeding cessation. *Journal of Human Lactation, 38*(1), 177–189. https://doi.org/10.1177/08903344211000284

Doan, T., Gardiner, A., Gay, C. L., & Lee, K. A. (2007). Breast-feeding increases sleep duration of new parents. *The Journal of Perinatal & Neonatal Nursing, 21*(3), 200–206. https://doi.org/10.1097/01.JPN.0000285809.36398.1b

Dodd, V., & Chalmers, C. (2003). Comparing the use of hydrogel dressings to lanolin ointment with lactating mothers. *Journal of Obstetric, Gynecologic, and Neonatal Nursing, 32*(4), 486–494. https://doi.org/10.1177/0884217503255098

Dørheim, S. K., Bondevik, G. T., Eberhard-Gran, M., & Bjorvatn, B. (2009a). Sleep and depression in postpartum women: A population-based study. *Sleep, 32*(7), 847–855. https://doi.org/10.1093/sleep/32.7.847

Dørheim, S. K., Bondevik, G. T., Eberhard-Gran, M., & Bjorvatn, B. (2009b). Subjective and objective sleep among depressed and non-depressed postnatal women. *Acta Psychiatrica Scandinavica, 119*(2), 128–136. https://doi.org/10.1111/j.1600-0447.2008.01272.x

Douglas, P. S., & Hill, P. S. (2013). Behavioral sleep interventions in the first six months of life do not improve outcomes for mothers or infants: A systematic review. *Journal of Developmental and Behavioral Pediatrics, 34*(7), 497–507. https://doi.org/10.1097/DBP.0b013e31829cafa6

Dugoua, J.-J., Mills, E., Perri, D., & Koren, G. (2006). Safety and efficacy of St. John's wort (hypericum) during pregnancy and lactation. *The Canadian Journal of Clinical Pharmacology, 13*(3), e268–e276.

Dunham, C. (1992). *Mamatoto: A celebration of birth.* Viking Penguin.

Dunstan, J. A., Mori, T. A., Barden, A., Beilin, L. J., Holt, P. G., Calder, P. C., Taylor, A. L., & Prescott, S. L. (2004). Effects of n-3 polyunsaturated fatty acid supplementation in pregnancy on maternal and fetal erythrocyte fatty acid composition. *European Journal of Clinical Nutrition, 58*(3), 429–437. https://doi.org/10.1038/sj.ejcn.1601825

Eberhard-Gran, M., Garthus-Niegel, S., Garthus-Niegel, K., & Eskild, A. (2010). Postnatal care: A cross-cultural and historical perspective. *Archives of Women's Mental Health, 13*(6), 459–466. https://doi.org/10.1007/s00737-010-0175-1

Edwards, R. C., Thullen, M. J., Korfmacher, J., Lantos, J. D., Henson, L. G., & Hans, S. L. (2013). Breastfeeding and complementary food: Randomized trial of community doula home visiting. *Pediatrics, 132*(Suppl. 2), S160–S166. https://doi.org/10.1542/peds.2013-1021P

Ekstrom, A. C., & Thorstensson, S. (2015). Nurses and midwives professional support increases with improved attitudes—Design and effects of a longitudinal randomized controlled process-oriented intervention. *BMC Pregnancy and Childbirth, 15*, 275. https://doi.org/10.1186/s12884-015-0712-z

Elmir, R., Schmied, V., Wilkes, L., & Jackson, D. (2010). Women's perceptions and experiences of a traumatic birth: A meta-ethnography. *Journal of Advanced Nursing, 66*(10), 2142–2153. https://doi.org/10.1111/j.1365-2648.2010.05391.x

Emery, C. F., Kiecolt-Glaser, J. K., Glaser, R., Malarkey, W. B., & Frid, D. J. (2005). Exercise accelerates wound healing among healthy older adults: A preliminary investigation. *The Journals of Gerontology: Series A. Biological Sciences and Medical Sciences, 60*(11), 1432–1436. https://doi.org/10.1093/gerona/60.11.1432

Emmott, E. H., Page, A. E., & Myers, S. (2020). Typologies of postnatal support and breastfeeding at two months in the UK. *Social Science & Medicine, 246*, 112791. https://doi.org/10.1016/j.socscimed.2020. 112791

Estrella, C. P., Mantaring, J. B. V., David, G. Z., & Taup, M. A. (2000). A double-blind, randomized controlled trial on the use of malunggay (*Moringa oleifera*) for augmentation of the volume of breastmilk among non-nursing mothers of preterm infants. *Philippine Journal of Medicine, 49*(1), 3–6.

Feldman-Winter, L., Szucs, K., Milano, A., Gottschlich, E., Sisk, B., & Schanler, R. J. (2017). National trends in pediatricians' practices and attitudes about breastfeeding: 1995 to 2014. *Pediatrics, 140*(4), e20171229. https://doi.org/10.1542/peds.2017-1229

Felitti, V. J., Anda, R. F., Nordenberg, D., Williamson, D. F., Spitz, A. M., Edwards, V., Koss, M. P., & Marks, J. S. (1998). Relationship of childhood abuse and household dysfunction to many of the leading causes of death in adults: The Adverse Childhood Experiences (ACE) Study. *American Journal of Preventive Medicine, 14*(4), 245–258. https:// doi.org/10.1016/S0749379798000178

Figley, C. (Ed.). (1986). *Trauma and its wake: Vol. 2. Traumatic stress theory, research, and intervention.* Bruner/Mazel.

Figueiredo, B., Dias, C. C., Brandão, S., Canário, C., & Nunes-Costa, R. (2013). Breastfeeding and postpartum depression: State of the art review. *Jornal de Pediatria, 89*(4), 332–338. https://doi.org/10.1016/ j.jped.2012.12.002

Figueiredo, B., Pinto, T. M., & Costa, R. (2021). Exclusive breastfeeding moderates the association between prenatal and postpartum depression. *Journal of Human Lactation, 37*(4), 784–794. https://doi.org/ 10.1177/0890334421991051

Galea, S., Vlahov, D., Resnick, H., Ahern, J., Susser, E., Gold, J., Bucuvalas, M., & Kilpatrick, D. (2003). Trends of probable post-traumatic stress disorder in New York City after the September 11 terrorist attacks.

American Journal of Epidemiology, 158(6), 514–524. https://doi.org/10.1093/aje/kwg187

Gao, L.-L., Xie, W., Yang, X., & Chan, S. W. (2015). Effects of an interpersonal-psychotherapy-oriented postnatal programme for Chinese first-time mothers: A randomized controlled trial. *International Journal of Nursing Studies, 52*(1), 22–29. https://doi.org/10.1016/j.ijnurstu.2014.06.006

Garbin, C. P., Sakalidis, V. S., Chadwick, L. M., Whan, E., Hartmann, P. E., & Geddes, D. T. (2013). Evidence of improved milk intake after frenotomy: A case report. *Pediatrics, 132*(5), e1413–e1417. https://doi.org/10.1542/peds.2012-2651

Garthus-Niegel, S., Horsch, A., Handtke, E., Von Soest, T., Ayers, S., Weidner, K., & Eberhard-Gran, M. (2018). The impact of postpartum posttraumatic stress and depression symptoms on couples' relationship satisfaction: A population-based prospective study. *Frontiers in Psychology, 9*. https://doi.org/10.3389/fpsyg.2018.01728

Gjerdingen, D. K., McGovern, P., Pratt, R., Johnson, L., & Crow, S. (2013). Postpartum doula and peer telephone support for postpartum depression: A pilot randomized controlled trial. *Journal of Primary Care & Community Health, 4*(1), 36–43. https://doi.org/10.1177/2150131912451598

Glaser, R., & Kiecolt-Glaser, J. K. (2005). Stress-induced immune dysfunction: Implications for health. *Nature Reviews: Immunology, 5*(3), 243–251. https://doi.org/10.1038/nri1571

Glover, R. (n.d.). *Rebecca Glover: Breastfeeding education materials.* https://www.rebeccaglover.com.au/

Goyal, D., Gay, C., & Lee, K. (2009). Fragmented maternal sleep is more strongly correlated with depressive symptoms than infant temperament at three months postpartum. *Archives of Women's Mental Health, 12*(4), 229–237. https://doi.org/10.1007/s00737-009-0070-9

Goyal, D., Gay, C. L., & Lee, K. A. (2007). Patterns of sleep disruption and depressive symptoms in new mothers. *The Journal of Perinatal & Neonatal Nursing, 21*(2), 123–129. https://doi.org/10.1097/01.JPN.0000270629.58746.96

Grajeda, R., & Pérez-Escamilla, R. (2002). Stress during labor and delivery is associated with delayed onset of lactation among urban Guatemalan women. *The Journal of Nutrition, 132*(10), 3055–3060. https://doi.org/10.1093/jn/131.10.3055

Grandjean, P., Bjerve, K. S., Weihe, P., & Steuerwald, U. (2001). Birthweight in a fishing community: Significance of essential fatty acids and marine food contaminants. *International Journal of Epidemiology, 30*(6), 1272–1278. https://doi.org/10.1093/ije/30.6.1272

Groer, M. W., & Davis, M. W. (2006). Cytokines, infections, stress, and dysphoric moods in breastfeeders and formula feeders. *Journal of Obstetric, Gynecologic, and Neonatal Nursing, 35*(5), 599–607. https://doi.org/10.1111/j.1552-6909.2006.00083.x

Groer, M. W., & Kendall-Tackett, K. A. (2011). *How breastfeeding protects women's health throughout the lifespan: The psychoneuroimmunology of human lactation.* Hale Publishing.

Hahn-Holbrook, J., Haselton, M. G., Dunkel Schetter, C., & Glynn, L. M. (2013). Does breastfeeding offer protection against maternal depressive symptomatology?: A prospective study from pregnancy to 2 years after birth. *Archives of Women's Mental Health, 16*(5), 411–422. https://doi.org/10.1007/s00737-013-0348-9

Hale, T. W. (2021). *Hale's medications and mothers' milk* (19th ed.). Springer Publishing.

Hale, T. W., Kendall-Tackett, K. A., & Cong, Z. (2018). Domperidone versus metoclopramide: Self-reported side effects in a large sample of breastfeeding mothers who used these medications to increase milk production. *Clinical Lactation, 9*(1), 10–17. https://doi.org/10.1891/2158-0782.9.1.10

Handlin, L., Jonas, W., Petersson, M., Ejdebäck, M., Ransjö-Arvidson, A.-B., Nissen, E., & Uvnäs-Moberg, K. (2009). Effects of sucking and skin-to-skin contact on maternal ACTH and cortisol levels during the second day postpartum-influence of epidural analgesia and oxytocin in the perinatal period. *Breastfeeding Medicine, 4*(4), 207–220. https://doi.org/10.1089/bfm.2009.0001

Heinrichs, M., Meinlschmidt, G., Neumann, I., Wagner, S., Kirschbaum, C., Ehlert, U., & Hellhammer, D. H. (2001). Effects of suckling on hypothalamic-pituitary-adrenal axis responses to psychosocial stress in postpartum lactating women. *The Journal of Clinical Endocrinology and Metabolism, 86*(10), 4798–4804. https://doi.org/10.1210/jcem.86.10.7919

Heise, A. M., & Wiessinger, D. (2011). Dysphoric milk ejection reflex: A case report. *International Breastfeeding Journal, 6*(6). https://doi.org/10.1186/1746-4358-6-6

Hibbeln, J. R. (2002). Seafood consumption, the DHA content of mothers' milk and prevalence rates of postpartum depression: A cross-national, ecological analysis. *Journal of Affective Disorders, 69*(1-3), 15–29. https://doi.org/10.1016/S0165-0327(01)00374-3

Hollister, S. (2018). *A lactation consultant's perspective on placenta encapsulation.* https://placentarisks.org/a-lactation-consultants-perspective-on-placenta-encapsulation/

Huang, L., Zhao, Y., Qiang, C., & Fan, B. (2018). Is cognitive behavioral therapy a better choice for women with postnatal depression? A systematic review and meta-analysis. *PLOS ONE, 13*(10), e0205243. https://doi.org/10.1371/journal.pone.0205243

Hughes, O., Mohamad, M. M., Doyle, P., & Burke, G. (2018). The significance of breastfeeding on sleep patterns during the first 48 hours postpartum for first time mothers. *Journal of Obstetrics & Gynaecology, 38*(3), 316–320. https://doi.org/10.1080/01443615.2017.1353594

Jones, I., & Craddock, N. (2001). Familiality of the puerperal trigger in bipolar disorder: Results of a family study. *The American Journal of Psychiatry, 158*(6), 913–917. https://doi.org/10.1176/appi.ajp.158.6.913

Jones, N. A., McFall, B. A., & Diego, M. A. (2004). Patterns of brain electrical activity in infants of depressed mothers who breastfeed and bottle feed: The mediating role of infant temperament. *Biological Psychology, 67*(1-2), 103–124. https://doi.org/10.1016/j.biopsycho.2004.03.010

Kendall-Tackett, K. (2007). A new paradigm for depression in new mothers: The central role of inflammation and how breastfeeding and anti-inflammatory treatments protect maternal mental health. *International Breastfeeding Journal, 2*(1), 6. https://doi.org/10.1186/1746-4358-2-6

Kendall-Tackett, K. A. (2010a). *Depression in new mothers: Causes, consequences and treatment options* (2nd ed.). Routledge.

Kendall-Tackett, K. (2010b). Long-chain omega-3 fatty acids and women's mental health in the perinatal period and beyond. *Journal of Midwifery & Women's Health, 55*(6), 561–567. https://doi.org/10.1016/j.jmwh.2010.02.014

Kendall-Tackett, K., Cong, Z., & Hale, T. W. (2013). Depression, sleep quality, and maternal well-being in postpartum women with a history of sexual assault: A comparison of breastfeeding, mixed-feeding, and formula-feeding mothers. *Breastfeeding Medicine, 8*(1), 16–22. https://doi.org/10.1089/bfm.2012.0024

Kendall-Tackett, K., Cong, Z., & Hale, T. (2018). The impact of feeding method and infant sleep location on mother/infant sleep, maternal depression, and mothers' well-being. *Clinical Lactation, 9*(3), 117–124. https://doi.org/10.1891/2158-0782.9.3.117

Kendall-Tackett, K. A. (2012). "Don't sleep with big knives": Interesting (and promising) developments in the mother–infant sleep debate. *Clinical Lactation, 3*(1), 9–12. https://doi.org/10.1891/215805312807010782

Kendall-Tackett, K. A. (2014). Childbirth-related posttraumatic stress disorder symptoms and implications for breastfeeding. *Clinical Lactation, 5*(2), 51–55. https://doi.org/10.1891/2158-0782.5.2.51

Kendall-Tackett, K. A. (2017). *Depression in new mothers* (3rd ed.). Routledge.

Kendall-Tackett, K. A., Cong, Z., & Hale, T. W. (2010). Mother–infant sleep locations and nighttime feeding behavior: U.S. data from the Survey of Mothers' Sleep and Fatigue. *Clinical Lactation, 1*(1), 27–31. https://doi.org/10.1891/215805310807011837

Kendall-Tackett, K. A., Cong, Z., & Hale, T. W. (2011). The effect of feeding method on sleep duration, maternal well-being, and postpartum depression. *Clinical Lactation, 2*(2), 22–26. https://doi.org/10.1891/215805311807011593

Kendall-Tackett, K. A., Cong, Z., & Hale, T. W. (2015). Birth interventions related to lower rates of exclusive breastfeeding and increased risk of postpartum depression in a large sample. *Clinical Lactation, 6*(3), 87–97. https://doi.org/10.1891/2158-0782.6.3.87

Kendall-Tackett, K. A., & Uvnas-Moberg, K. (2018). A response to Heise and Wiessinger. *Clinical Lactation, 9*(3), 106–107. https://doi.org/10.1891/2158-0782.9.3.106

Kendall-Tackett, K. A., Walker, M., & Genna, C. W. (Eds.). (2018). *Tongue-tie: Expert roundtable.* Praeclarus Press.

Khan, T. V., & Ritchie, J. (2019). Management of common breastfeeding problems: Nipple pain and infections. In K. A. Kendall-Tackett (Ed.), *Breast and nipple pain II* (pp. 121–140). Praeclarus Press.

Kiecolt-Glaser, J. K., Belury, M. A., Porter, K., Beversdorf, D. Q., Lemeshow, S., & Glaser, R. (2007). Depressive symptoms, omega-6:omega-3 fatty acids, and inflammation in older adults. *Psychosomatic Medicine, 69*(3), 217–224. https://doi.org/10.1097/PSY.0b013e3180313a45

Kiecolt-Glaser, J. K., Christian, L., Preston, H., Houts, C. R., Malarkey, W. B., Emery, C. F., & Glaser, R. (2010). Stress, inflammation, and yoga practice. *Psychosomatic Medicine, 72*(2), 113–121. https://doi.org/10.1097/PSY.0b013e3181cb9377

Kiecolt-Glaser, J. K., Derry, H. M., & Fagundes, C. P. (2015). Inflammation: Depression fans the flames and feasts on the heat. *The American Journal of Psychiatry, 172*(11), 1075–1091. https://doi.org/10.1176/appi.ajp.2015.15020152

Kim, Y.-D., Heo, I., Shin, B.-C., Crawford, C., Kang, H.-W., & Lim, J.-H. (2013). Acupuncture for posttraumatic stress disorder: A systematic review of randomized controlled trials and prospective clinical trials. *Evidence-Based Complementary and Alternative Medicine, 2013*, 615857. https://doi.org/10.1155/2013/615857

Klier, C. M., Schäfer, M. R., Schmid-Siegel, B., Lenz, G., & Mannel, M. (2002). St. John's wort (*Hypericum perforatum*)—Is it safe during breastfeeding? *Pharmacopsychiatry, 35*(1), 29–30. https://doi.org/10.1055/s-2002-19832

Kozhimannil, K. B., Jou, J., Attanasio, L. B., Joarnt, L. K., & McGovern, P. (2014). Medically complex pregnancies and early breastfeeding behaviors: A retrospective analysis. *PLOS ONE, 9*(8), e104820. https://doi.org/10.1371/journal.pone.0104820

Lahr, M. B., Rosenberg, K. D., & Lapidus, J. A. (2005). Bedsharing and maternal smoking in a population-based survey of new mothers. *Pediatrics, 116*(4), e530–e542. https://doi.org/10.1542/peds.2005-0354

Lahr, M. B., Rosenberg, K. D., & Lapidus, J. A. (2007). Maternal–infant bedsharing: Risk factors for bedsharing in a population-based survey of new mothers and implications for SIDS risk reduction. *Maternal and Child Health Journal, 11*(3), 277–286. https://doi.org/10.1007/s10995-006-0166-z

Lavigne, V. (2016). Lactation consultants' perceptions of musculoskeletal disorder affecting breastfeeding. *Clinical Lactation, 7*(1), 30–36. https://doi.org/10.1891/2158-0782.7.1.30

Lawvere, S., & Mahoney, M. C. (2005). St. John's wort. *American Family Physician, 72*(11), 2249–2254.

Leviniene, G., Tamulevičienė, E., Kudzyte, J., Petrauskiene, A., Zaborskis, A., Aželiene, I., & Labanauskas, L. (2013). Factors associated with breastfeeding duration. *Medicina, 49*(9), 415–421.

Li, R., Fein, S. B., & Grummer-Strawn, L. M. (2010). Do infants fed from bottles lack self-regulation of milk intake compared with directly breastfed infants? *Pediatrics*, *125*(6), e1386–e1393. https://doi.org/10.1542/peds.2009-2549

Li, S., Zhong, W., Peng, W., & Jiang, G. (2018). Effectiveness of acupuncture in postpartum depression: A systematic review and meta-analysis. *Acupuncture in Medicine*, *36*(5), 295–301. https://doi.org/10.1136/acupmed-2017-011530

Lukas, C. (2019). *One in four women go to work two weeks after giving birth.* https://www.forbes.com/sites/carrielukas/2019/12/13/one-in-four-women-dont-go-to-work-two-weeks-after-giving-birth/?sh=7df1f8227a61

Maes, M., Christophe, A., Bosmans, E., Lin, A., & Neels, H. (2000). In humans, serum polyunsaturated fatty acid levels predict the response of proinflammatory cytokines to psychologic stress. *Biological Psychiatry*, *47*(10), 910–920. https://doi.org/10.1016/S0006-3223(99)00268-1

Maes, M., Verkerk, R., Bonaccorso, S., Ombelet, W., Bosmans, E., & Scharpé, S. (2002). Depressive and anxiety symptoms in the early puerperium are related to increased degradation of tryptophan into kynurenine, a phenomenon which is related to immune activation. *Life Sciences*, *71*(16), 1837–1848. https://doi.org/10.1016/S0024-3205(02)01853-2

Manber, R., Schnyer, R. N., Allen, J. J. B., Rush, A. J., & Blasey, C. M. (2004). Acupuncture: A promising treatment for depression during pregnancy. *Journal of Affective Disorders*, *83*(1), 89–95. https://doi.org/10.1016/j.jad.2004.05.009

Manber, R., Schnyer, R. N., Lyell, D., Chambers, A. S., Caughey, A. B., Druzin, M., Carlyle, E., Celio, C., Gress, J. L., Huang, M. I., Kalista, T., Martin-Okada, R., & Allen, J. J. B. (2010). Acupuncture for depression during pregnancy: A randomized controlled trial [erratum at https://doi.org/10.3410/f.2274991.1895097]. *Obstetrics and Gynecology*, *115*(3), 511–520. https://doi.org/10.1097/AOG.0b013e3181cc0816

Mannel, R., & Mannel, R. S. (2006). Staffing for hospital lactation programs: Recommendations from a tertiary care teaching hospital. *Journal of Human Lactation*, *22*(4), 409–417. https://doi.org/10.1177/0890334406294166

Marasco, L., & West, D. (2019). *Making more milk: The breastfeeding guide to increasing your milk production* (2nd ed.). McGraw-Hill.

Markhus, M. W., Skotheim, S., Graff, I. E., Frøyland, L., Braarud, H. C., Stormark, K. M., & Malde, M. K. (2013). Low omega-3 index in pregnancy is a possible biological risk factor for postpartum depression. *PLOS ONE, 8*(7), e67617. https://doi.org/10.1371/journal.pone.0067617

Martin, K. (2011). A time and place to pump: What lactation consultants need to know about the few federal protections for employed breastfeeding mothers. *Clinical Lactation, 2*(2), 20–21. https://doi.org/10.1891/215805311807011647

Matthews, G. (1987). *"Just a housewife": The rise and fall of domesticity in America*. Oxford University Press.

Matthiesen, A., Ransjo-Arvidson, A.-B., Nissen, E., & Uvnäs-Moberg, K. (2001). Postpartum maternal oxytocin release by newborns: Effect of infant hand massage and sucking. *Birth, 28*(1), 13–19. https://doi.org/10.1046/j.1523-536x.2001.00013.x

McGovern, P., Dowd, B., Gjerdingen, D., Gross, C. R., Kenney, S., Ukestad, L., McCaffrey, D., & Lundberg, U. (2006). Postpartum health of employed mothers 5 weeks after childbirth. *Annals of Family Medicine, 4*(2), 159–167. https://doi.org/10.1370/afm.519

McKenna, J. J. (2020). *Safe infant sleep: Expert answers to your cosleeping questions*. Platypus Media.

McKenna, J. J., & Volpe, L. E. (2007). Sleeping with baby: An Internet-based sampling of parental experiences, choices, perceptions, and interpretations in a Western Industrialized context. *Infant and Child Development, 16*(4), 359–385. https://doi.org/10.1002/icd.525

McLeish, J., & Redshaw, M. (2019). "Being the best person that they can be and the best mum": A qualitative study of community volunteer doula support for disadvantaged mothers before and after birth in England. *BMC Pregnancy and Childbirth, 19*(1), 21. https://doi.org/10.1186/s12884-018-2170-x

Middlemiss, W., Granger, D. A., Goldberg, W. A., & Nathans, L. (2011). Asynchrony of mother–infant hypothalamic–pituitary–adrenal axis activity following extinction of infant responses induced during the transition to sleep. *Early Human Development, 88*(4), 227–232. https://doi.org/10.1016/j.earlhumdev.2011.08.010

Middlemiss, W., & Kendall-Tackett, K. A. (Eds.). (2014). *The science of mother–infant sleep: Current findings on bedsharing, breastfeeding, sleep training, and normal infant sleep*. Praeclarus Press.

Middlemiss, W., Stevens, H., Ridgway, L., McDonald, S., & Koussa, M. (2017). Response-based sleep intervention: Helping infants sleep without making them cry. *Early Human Development, 108,* 49–57. https://doi.org/10.1016/j.earlhumdev.2017.03.008

Middleton, P., Gomersall, J. C., Gould, J. F., Shepherd, E., Olsen, S. F., & Makrides, M. (2018). Omega-3 fatty acid addition during pregnancy [erratum at https://doi.org/10.1002/14651858.CD003402.pub2]. *Cochrane Database of Systematic Reviews,* (11):CD003402. https://doi.org/10.1002/14651858.CD003402.pub3

Milinco, M., Travan, L., Cattaneo, A., Knowles, A., Sola, M. V., Causin, E., Cortivo, C., Degrassi, M., Di Tommaso, F., Verardi, G., Dipietro, L., Piazza, M., Scolz, S., Rossetto, M., Ronfani, L., & the Trieste BN (Biological Nurturing) Investigators. (2020). Effectiveness of biological nurturing on early breastfeeding problems: A randomized controlled trial. *International Breastfeeding Journal, 15*(1), 21. https://doi.org/10.1186/s13006-020-00261-4

Miller, J. (2019). *Evidence-based chiropractic care for infants: Rationale, therapies, and outcomes.* Praeclarus Press.

Miller, J. (2020). Breastfeeding support team: When to add a chiropractor. *Clinical Lactation, 11*(1), 7–20. https://doi.org/10.1891/2158-0782.11.1.7

Mocking, R. J. T., Steijn, K., Roos, C., Assies, J., Bergink, V., Ruhe, H. G., & Schene, A. H. (2020). Omega-3 fatty acid supplementation for perinatal depression: A meta-analysis. *Journal of Clinical Psychiatry, 81*(5), 19r13195. https://doi.org/10.4088/JCP.19r13106

Modarres, M., Afrasiabi, S., Rahnama, P., & Montazeri, A. (2012). Prevalence and risk factors of childbirth-related post-traumatic stress symptoms. *BMC Pregnancy and Childbirth, 12*(1), 88. https://doi.org/10.1186/1471-2393-12-88

Mohrbacher, N. S., & Kendall-Tackett, K. A. (2010). *Breastfeeding made simple: Seven natural laws for nursing mothers* (2nd ed.). New Harbinger Publications.

Morton, C. H., & Clift, E. G. (2014). *Birth ambassadors: Doula and the re-emergence of woman-supported birth in America.* Praeclarus Press.

Nakamura, A., van der Waerden, J., Melchior, M., Bolze, C., El-Khoury, F., & Pryor, L. (2019). Physical activity during pregnancy and postpartum depression: Systematic review and meta-analysis. *Journal of Affective Disorders, 246,* 29–41. https://doi.org/10.1016/j.jad.2018.12.009

Narvaez, D. (2013). The dangers of "crying it out": Damaging children and their relationships for the long-term. In W. Middlemiss & K. A. Kendall-Tackett (Eds.), *The science of mother–infant sleep: Current findings on bedsharing, breastfeeding, sleep training, and normal infant sleep* (pp. 97–106). Praeclarus Press.

Needels, M. S. (2019). Education is key for increasing breastfeeding duration among working mothers. *Clinical Lactation, 10*(3), 121–126. https://doi.org/10.1891/2158-0782.10.3.121

Newman, J. (n.d.-a). *All-purpose nipple ointment.* https://ibconline.ca/information-sheets/all-purpose-nipple-ointment-apno/

Newman, J. (n.d.-b). *Herbal remedies for milk supply.* https://ibconline.ca/information-sheets/herbal-remedies-for-milk-supply/

Ngoenthong, P., Sansiriphun, N., Fongkaew, W., & Chaloumsuk, N. (2020). Integrative review of fathers' perspectives on breastfeeding support. *Journal of Obstetric, Gynecologic, and Neonatal Nursing, 49*(1), 16–26. https://doi.org/10.1016/j.jogn.2019.09.005

Nicholson, B., & Parker, L. (2019). *Attached at the heart: Eight proven parenting principles for raising connected and compassionate children.* Praeclarus Press.

Norman, E., Sherburn, M., Osborne, R. H., & Galea, M. P. (2010). An exercise and education program improves well-being of new mothers: A randomized controlled trial. *Physical Therapy, 90*(3), 348–355. https://doi.org/10.2522/ptj.20090139

Oddy, W. H., Kendall, G. E., Li, J., Jacoby, P., Robinson, M., de Klerk, N. H., Silburn, S. R., Zubrick, S. R., Landau, L. I., & Stanley, F. J. (2010). The long-term effects of breastfeeding on child and adolescent mental health: A pregnancy cohort study followed for 14 years. *The Journal of Pediatrics, 156*(4), 568–574. https://doi.org/10.1016/j.jpeds.2009.10.020

Oparah, J. C., Arega, H., Hudson, D., Jones, L., & Oseguera, T. (2018). *Battling over birth: Black women and the maternal health care crisis.* Praeclarus Press.

Owenz, M. (2021). *Spoiled right: Delaying screens and giving children what they really need.* Praeclarus Press.

Park, S., & Choi, N.-K. (2019). Breastfeeding reduces risk of depression later in life in the postmenopausal period: A Korean population-based study. *Journal of Affective Disorders, 248*(1), 13–17. https://doi.org/10.1016/j.jad.2018.12.081

Pearson, A. (2002). *I don't know how she does it: The life of Kate Reddy, working mother.* Anchor.

Pennebaker, J. (2004). *Writing to heal: A guided journal for recovering from trauma and emotional upheaval.* Center for Journal Therapy.

Peterson, M. (2016). *Seven sisters for seven days: The mothers' manual for community-based postpartum care.* Praeclarus Press.

Prentice, J. C., Lu, M. C., Lange, L., & Halfon, N. (2002). The association between reported childhood sexual abuse and breastfeeding initiation. *Journal of Human Lactation, 18*(3), 219–226. https://doi.org/10.1177/089033440201800303

Price, A. M. H., Wake, M., Ukoumunne, O. C., & Hiscock, H. (2012). Five-year follow-up of harms and benefits of behavioral infant sleep intervention: Randomized trial. *Pediatrics, 130*(4), 643–651. https://doi.org/10.1542/peds.2011-3467

Pritchett, R. V., Daley, A. J., & Jolly, K. (2017). Does aerobic exercise reduce postpartum depressive symptoms? A systematic review and meta-analysis. *The British Journal of General Practice, 67*(663), e684–e691. https://doi.org/10.3399/bjgp17X692525

Puig, J., Englund, M. M., Simpson, J. A., & Collins, W. A. (2013). Predicting adult physical illness from infant attachment: A prospective longitudinal study. *Health Psychology, 32*(4), 409–417. https://doi.org/10.1037/a0028889

Putnam, R. D. (2000). *Bowling alone: The collapse and revival of American community.* Simon & Schuster.

Quinn, T. J., & Carey, G. B. (1999). Does exercise intensity or diet influence lactic acid accumulation in breast milk? *Medicine and Science in Sports and Exercise, 31*(1), 105–110. https://doi.org/10.1097/00005768-199901000-00017

Ram, K. T., Bobby, P., Hailpern, S. M., Lo, J. C., Schocken, M., Skurnick, J., & Santoro, N. (2008). Duration of lactation is associated with lower prevalence of the metabolic syndrome in midlife—SWAN, the Study of Women's Health Across the Nation. *American Journal of Obstetrics and Gynecology, 198*(3), 268.e1–268.e6. https://doi.org/10.1016/j.ajog.2007.11.044

Raphael, D. (1955). *The tender gift: Breastfeeding.* Schocken.

Rich-Edwards, J. W., James-Todd, T., Mohllajee, A., Kleinman, K., Burke, A., Gillman, M. W., & Wright, R. J. (2011). Lifetime maternal experiences of abuse and risk of pre-natal depression in two demographically distinct populations in Boston. *International Journal of Epidemiology*, *40*(2), 375–384. https://doi.org/10.1093/ije/dyq247

Rich-Edwards, J. W., Spiegelman, D., Lividoti Hibert, E. N., Jun, H.-J., Todd, T. J., Kawachi, I., & Wright, R. J. (2010). Abuse in childhood and adolescence as a predictor of Type 2 diabetes in adult women. *American Journal of Preventive Medicine*, *39*(6), 529–536. https://doi.org/10.1016/j.amepre.2010.09.007

Righard, L., & Alade, M. O. (1990). Effect of delivery room routines on success of first breast-feed. *Lancet*, *336*(8723), 1105–1107. https://doi.org/10.1016/0140-6736(90)92579-7

Robinson, M., Whitehouse, A. J. O., Newnham, J. P., Gorman, S., Jacoby, P., Holt, B. J., Serralha, M., Tearne, J. E., Holt, P. G., Hart, P. H., & Kusel, M. M. H. (2014). Low maternal serum vitamin D during pregnancy and the risk for postpartum depression symptoms [erratum at https://doi.org/10.3410/f.718324433.793532167]. *Archives of Women's Mental Health*, *17*(3), 213–219. https://doi.org/10.1007/s00737-014-0422-y

Rowlands, I. J., & Redshaw, M. (2012). Mode of birth and women's psychological and physical wellbeing in the postnatal period. *BMC Pregnancy and Childbirth*, *12*(1), 138. https://doi.org/10.1186/1471-2393-12-138

Ruddle, L. (2020). *Relactation: A guide to rebuilding your milk supply*. Praeclarus Press.

Ruddle, L. (2021). *Mixed-up: Combination feeding by necessity or choice*. Praeclarus Press.

Rupke, S. J., Blecke, D., & Renfrow, M. (2006). Cognitive therapy for depression. *American Family Physician*, *73*(1), 83–86.

Sanford, D. (2018). *Stress less, live better: Five simple steps to ease anxiety, worry, and self-criticism*. Praeclarus Press.

Sanford, D. (2019). *Stress less, live better: For pregnancy, postpartum, and early motherhood*. Praeclarus Press.

Sapolsky, R. M. (1996). Why stress is bad for your brain. *Science*, *273*(5276), 749–750. https://doi.org/10.1126/science.273.5276.749

Schiepers, O. J., Wichers, M. C., & Maes, M. (2005). Cytokines and major depression. *Progress in Neuro-Psychopharmacology & Biological Psychiatry*, *29*(2), 201–217. https://doi.org/10.1016/j.pnpbp.2004.11.003

Schnell, A. (2013). *Breastfeeding without birthing: A breastfeeding guide for mothers through adoption, surrogacy, and other special circumstances.* Praeclarus Press.

Schore, A. N. (2000). Attachment and the regulation of the right brain. *Attachment and Human Development, 2*(1), 23–47. https://doi.org/10.1080/146167300361309

Schore, A. N. (2001). Effects of a secure attachment relationship on right brain development, affect regulation, and infant mental health. *Infant Mental Health Journal, 22*(1-2), 7–66. https://doi.org/10.1002/1097-0355(200101/04)22:1<7::AID-IMHJ2>3.0.CO;2-N

Schore, A. N. (2009). Relational trauma and the developing right brain: An interface of psychoanalytic self psychology and neuroscience. *Annals of the New York Academy of Sciences, 1159*(1), 189–203. https://doi.org/10.1111/j.1749-6632.2009.04474.x

Schulz, V. (2006). Safety of St. John's wort extract compared to synthetic antidepressants. *Phytomedicine, 13*(3), 199–204. https://doi.org/10.1016/j.phymed.2005.07.005

Schwarz, E. B., Ray, R. M., Stuebe, A. M., Allison, M. A., Ness, R. B., Freiberg, M. S., & Cauley, J. A. (2009). Duration of lactation and risk factors for maternal cardiovascular disease. *Obstetrics and Gynecology, 113*(5), 974–982. https://doi.org/10.1097/01.AOG.0000346884.67796.ca

Shaw, J. G., Asch, S. M., Kimerling, R., Frayne, S. M., Shaw, K. A., & Phibbs, C. S. (2014). Posttraumatic stress disorder and risk of spontaneous preterm birth. *Obstetrics and Gynecology, 124*(6), 1111–1119. https://doi.org/10.1097/AOG.0000000000000542

Shen, Y., Leng, J., Li, W., Zhang, S., Liu, H., Shao, P., Wang, P., Wang, L., Tian, H., Zhang, C., Yang, X., Yu, Z., Hou, L., Tuomilehto, J., & Hu, G. (2019). Lactation intensity and duration to postpartum diabetes and prediabetes risk in women with gestational diabetes. *Diabetes/Metabolism Research and Reviews, 35*(3), e3115. https://doi.org/10.1002/dmrr.3115

Shields, B. (2005). *Down came the rain: My journey through postpartum depression.* Hyperion.

Shonkoff, J. P., Boyce, W. T., & McEwen, B. S. (2009). Neuroscience, molecular biology, and the childhood roots of health disparities: Building a new framework for health promotion and disease prevention. *Journal of the American Medical Association, 301*(21), 2252–2259. https://doi.org/10.1001/jama.2009.754

Simpson, M., & Catling, C. (2016). Understanding psychological traumatic birth experiences: A literature review. *Women and Birth, 29*(3), 203–207. https://doi.org/10.1016/j.wombi.2015.10.009

Söderquist, J., Wijma, B., Thorbert, G., & Wijma, K. (2009). Risk factors in pregnancy for post-traumatic stress and depression after childbirth. *British Journal of Obstetrics and Gynaecology, 116*(5), 672–680. https://doi.org/10.1111/j.1471-0528.2008.02083.x

Sørbø, M. F., Lukasse, M., Brantsaeter, A. L., & Grimstad, H. (2015). Past and recent abuse is associated with early cessation of breast feeding: Results from a large prospective cohort in Norway. *BMJ Open, 5*(12), 009240. https://doi.org/10.1136/bmjopen-2015-009240

Speisman, B. B., Storch, E. A., & Abramowitz, J. S. (2011). Postpartum obsessive-compulsive disorder. *Journal of Obstetric, Gynecologic, and Neonatal Nursing, 40*(6), 680–690. https://doi.org/10.1111/j.1552-6909.2011.01294.x

Sriraman, N. K., Evans, A. E., Lawrence, R., Noble, L., & the Academy of Breastfeeding Medicine's Board of Directors. (2018). Academy of Breastfeeding Medicine's 2017 position statement on informal breast milk sharing for the term healthy infant. *Breastfeeding Medicine, 13*(1), 2–4. https://doi.org/10.1089/bfm.2017.29064.nks

Starkweather, A. R. (2007). The effects of exercise on perceived stress and IL-6 levels among older adults. *Biological Research for Nursing, 8*(3), 186–194. https://doi.org/10.1177/1099800406295990

Stern, G., & Kruckman, L. (1983). Multi-disciplinary perspectives on postpartum depression: An anthropological critique. *Social Science & Medicine, 17*(15), 1027–1041. https://doi.org/10.1016/0277-9536(83)90408-2

Stramrood, C. A. I., Paarlberg, K. M., Huis In 't Veld, E. M. J., Berger, L. W. A. R., Vingerhoets, A. J. J. M., Schultz, W. C. M. W., & van Pampus, M. G. (2011). Posttraumatic stress following childbirth in homelike- and hospital settings. *Journal of Psychosomatic Obstetrics and Gynaecology, 32*(2), 88–97. https://doi.org/10.3109/0167482X.2011.569801

Strathearn, L., Mamun, A. A., Najman, J. M., & O'Callaghan, M. J. (2009). Does breastfeeding protect against substantiated child abuse and neglect? A 15-year cohort study. *Pediatrics, 123*(2), 483–493. https://doi.org/10.1542/peds.2007-3546

Stuebe, A. M., Rich-Edwards, J. W., Willett, W. C., Manson, J. E., & Michels, K. B. (2005). Duration of lactation and incidence of type 2 diabetes.

Journal of the American Medical Association, 294(20), 2601–2610. https://doi.org/10.1001/jama.294.20.2601

Su, D., Zhao, Y., Binns, C., Scott, J., & Oddy, W. (2007). Breast-feeding mothers can exercise: Results of a cohort study. *Public Health Nutrition, 10*(10), 1089–1093. https://doi.org/10.1017/S1368980007699534

Tappin, D., Ecob, R., & Brooke, H. (2005). Bedsharing, roomsharing, and sudden infant death syndrome in Scotland: A case–control study. *The Journal of Pediatrics, 147*(1), 32–37. https://doi.org/10.1016/j.jpeds.2005.01.035

Taylor, A., & Parekh, J. (2020). Follow-up care for the healthy newborn. In T. K. McInerny, H. M. Adam, D. E. Campbell, T. G. DeWitt, J. M. Foy, & D. M. Kamat (Eds.), *American Academy of Pediatrics textbook of pediatric care* (pp. 790–796). American Academy of Pediatrics.

Teychenne, M., & York, R. (2013). Physical activity, sedentary behavior, and postnatal depressive symptoms: A review. *American Journal of Preventive Medicine, 45*(2), 217–227. https://doi.org/10.1016/j.amepre.2013.04.004

Uchino, B. N., Trettevik, R., Kent de Grey, R. G., Cronan, S., Hogan, J., & Baucom, B. R. W. (2018). Social support, social integration, and inflammatory cytokines: A meta-analysis. *Health Psychology, 37*(5), 462–471. https://doi.org/10.1037/hea0000594

Ukah, U. V., Adu, P. A., De Silva, D. A., & von Dadelszen, P. (2016). The impact of history of adverse childhood experiences on breastfeeding initiation and exclusivity: Findings from a National Population Health Survey. *Breastfeeding Medicine, 11*(10), 544–550. https://doi.org/10.1089/bfm.2016.0053

U.S. Department of Labor. (n.d.). *Section 7(r) of the Fair Labor Standards Act—Break time for nursing mothers provision.* https://www.dol.gov/agencies/whd/nursing-mothers/law

U.S. Lactation Consultant Association. (2020). *Who's who? An at-a-glance look at lactation support in the United States.* https://uslca.org/wp-content/uploads/2015/05/Whos-Who-Short1.pdf

U.S. Office of Personnel Management. (n.d.). *Child care resources handbook.* https://www.opm.gov/policy-data-oversight/worklife/reference-materials/child-care-resources-handbook/#:~:text=Staff%2FChild%20Ratios%20at%20Child%20Care%20Centers&text=For%20infants%20(birth%2D15%20months,children%20(1%3A4)

U.S. Office of Women's Health. (n.d.). *Business case for breastfeeding: For business managers.* https://www.womenshealth.gov/files/documents/bcfb_business-case-for-breastfeeding-for-business-managers.pdf

U.S. Office of Women's Health. (2018). *Business case for breastfeeding.* https://www.womenshealth.gov/breastfeeding/breastfeeding-home-work-and-public/breastfeeding-and-going-back-work/business-case

Uvnäs Moberg, K. (2013). *The hormone of closeness: The role of oxytocin in relationships.* Pinter & Martin.

Uvnäs Moberg, K. (2015). *Oxytocin: The biological guide to motherhood.* Praeclarus Press.

Uvnäs Moberg, K., Ekström-Bergström, A., Buckley, S., Massarotti, C., Pajalic, Z., Luegmair, K., Kotlowska, A., Lengler, L., Olza, I., Grylka-Baeschlin, S., Leahy-Warren, P., Hadjigeorgiu, E., Villarmea, S., & Dencker, A. (2020). Maternal plasma levels of oxytocin during breastfeeding—A systematic review. *PLOS ONE, 15*(8), e0235806. https://doi.org/10.1371/journal.pone.0235806

Uvnäs Moberg, K., & Kendall-Tackett, K. A. (2018). The mystery of D-MER: What can hormonal research tell us about dysphoric milk-ejection reflex? *Clinical Lactation, 9*(1), 23–29. https://doi.org/10.1891/2158-0782.9.1.23

van Gurp, G., Meterissian, G. B., Haiek, L. N., McCusker, J., & Bellavance, F. (2002). St John's wort or sertraline? Randomized controlled trial in primary care. *Canadian Family Physician, 48*, 905–912.

Vennemann, M. M., Bajanowski, T., Brinkmann, B., Jorch, G., Yücesan, K., Sauerland, C., Mitchell, E. A., & the GeSID Study Group. (2009). Does breastfeeding reduce the risk of sudden infant death syndrome? *Pediatrics, 123*(3), e406–e410. https://doi.org/10.1542/peds.2008-2145

Vennemann, M. M., Hense, H.-W., Bajanowski, T., Blair, P. S., Complojer, C., Moon, R. Y., & Kiechl-Kohlendorfer, U. (2012). Bed sharing and the risk of sudden infant death syndrome: Can we resolve the debate? *The Journal of Pediatrics, 160*(1), 44–48.e2. https://doi.org/10.1016/j.jpeds.2011.06.052

Wagner, C. L., Taylor, S. N., & Hollis, B. (2010). *New insights into Vitamin D during pregnancy, lactation, and early infancy.* Hale Publishing.

Walker, M. (2018). Is exclusive breastfeeding dangerous? *Clinical Lactation, 9*(4), 171–182. https://doi.org/10.1891/2158-0782.9.4.171

Walker, M. (2020). *Breastfeeding the late preterm infant.* Praeclarus Press.

Watkins, S., Meltzer-Brody, S., Zolnoun, D., & Stuebe, A. (2011). Early breastfeeding experiences and postpartum depression. *Obstetrics and Gynecology, 118*(2 Pt. 1), 214–221. https://doi.org/10.1097/AOG.0b013e3182260a2d

Webber, S. (1992). Supporting the postpartum family. *The Doula, 23,* 16–17.

Webber, S. (2012). *The gentle art of newborn family care.* Praeclarus Press.

West, D. (2001). *Defining your own success: Breastfeeding after breast reduction.* La Leche League International.

Wiessinger, D. (1998). A breastfeeding teaching tool using a sandwich analogy for latch-on. *Journal of Human Lactation, 14*(1), 51–56. https://doi.org/10.1177/089033449801400116

Wilson-Clay, B., & Hoover, K. (2017). *Breastfeeding atlas* (6th ed.). LactNews Press.

World Health Organization. (n.d.). *Ten steps to successful breastfeeding.* https://www.who.int/activities/promoting-baby-friendly-hospitals/ten-steps-to-successful-breastfeeding

Yusuff, A. S. M., Tang, L., Binns, C. W., & Lee, A. H. (2016). Breastfeeding and postnatal depression: A prospective cohort study in Sabah, Malaysia. *Journal of Human Lactation, 32*(2), 277–281. https://doi.org/10.1177/0890334415620788

Zhang, B. Z., Zhang, H. Y., Liu, H. H., Li, H. J., & Wang, J. S. (2015). Breastfeeding and maternal hypertension and diabetes: A population-based cross-sectional study. *Breastfeeding Medicine, 10*(3), 163–167. https://doi.org/10.1089/bfm.2014.0116

Zlotnick, C., Miller, I. W., Pearlstein, T., Howard, M., & Sweeney, P. (2006). A preventive intervention for pregnant women on public assistance at risk for postpartum depression. *The American Journal of Psychiatry, 163*(8), 1443–1445. https://doi.org/10.1176/ajp.2006.163.8.1443

INDEX

ABOUT THE AUTHOR

Kathleen Kendall-Tackett, PhD, IBCLC, FAPA, is a health psychologist and international board certified lactation consultant (IBCLC). She is a Fellow of the American Psychological Association (APA) in health and trauma psychology. Dr. Kendall-Tackett was trained as a researcher in family violence and sexual assault and also specializes in perinatal mental illness. She was a founder and past president of the APA's Division of Trauma Psychology and is currently chair-elect of the APA Publications and Communications Board that oversees all APA books and journals.

Dr. Kendall-Tackett has been an accredited La Leche League leader since 1994 and has served in many capacities on boards and in leadership positions within the breastfeeding world. She became an IBCLC in 2002. Dr. Kendall-Tackett started working with breastfeeding mothers as a volunteer, which was supposed to be the happy counterpart to her trauma and depression work. However, she was soon asked to speak at breastfeeding conferences on depression, trauma, and sexual assault and has been doing that ever since. She has been invited to speak in 49 U.S. states, across Canada, and in 15 other countries. For many years, she was the only psychologist happily occupying the space between lactation and psychology, but is delighted that younger colleagues have taken up the torch.

Dr. Kendall-Tackett was the founding editor-in-chief of the U.S. Lactation Consultant Association's journal, *Clinical Lactation*, a position she held for 11 years. For the past 8 years, she has been editor-in-chief for the APA journal *Psychological Trauma*. For 6 years, she edited both journals at the same time. Dr. Kendall-Tackett is the author 490 articles and the author or editor of 40 books, including the bestselling *Breastfeeding Made Simple* (with Nancy Mohrbacher) and the Clinical Lactation Monograph Series.

A full-time book editor since 2008, Dr. Kendall-Tackett formed her own publishing company, Praeclarus Press, in 2011, which specializes in women's health. Both of her adult sons work with her and her team, and they publish amazing books, webinars, and art. To find out more, go to https://www.PraeclarusPress.com.

Dr. Kendall-Tackett lives in Amarillo, Texas, with her husband, Doug, and an entire herd of cats and dogs. She enjoys Irish music and red-dirt country, travel photography, and singing with the Amarillo Master Chorale. She continues to write and speak at live events and webinars in the United States, Canada, Europe, Australia, and New Zealand. Her schedule of upcoming events and online education is available at https://www.KathleenKendall-Tackett.com.